FRCR Physics Notes

This title is available in paperback and as an e-book.

For more details, please see
www.radiologycafe.com/frcr-physics-notes
or scan this QR code:

FRCR Physics Notes

Dr Sarah Abdulla

MBBS MA(Cantab) FRCR PGCert

Consultant Neuroradiologist

Salford Royal NHS Foundation Trust

Dr Christopher Clarke

MBChB FRCR

Consultant Gastrointestinal and Hepatobiliary Radiologist

Nottingham University Hospitals NHS Trust

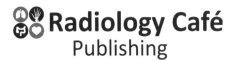 **Radiology Café**
Publishing

ISBN: 978-1-9999885-2-4 (paperback) | 978-1-9999885-3-1 (epub)

Illustrations by Sarah Abdulla.

Cover design by Christopher Clarke.

v

Contents

Preface   vii
Acknowledgements   ix

Chapter 1   Basic Science

1.1   Atomic Structure   3
1.2   Electromagnetic Radiation   6
1.3   Radioactive Decay   10

Chapter 2   X-Ray Imaging

2.1   Production of X-Rays   17
2.2   Interaction with Matter   27
2.3   Digital Radiography   34
2.4   Image Quality   43
2.5   Quality Assurance   53
2.6   Mammography   59
2.7   Fluoroscopy   65

Chapter 3   CT Imaging

3.1   CT Equipment   79
3.2   Acquiring an Image (Part 1)   85
3.3   Acquiring an Image (Part 2)   90
3.4   Dual-Energy CT   93
3.5   CT Image Quality   97
3.6   CT Artefacts   103
3.7   CT Dose   110

Chapter 4   Ultrasound Imaging

4.1   Properties of Sound   115
4.2   Ultrasound Machine   119
4.3   Producing an Ultrasound Beam   123
4.4   Image Properties   127
4.5   Doppler   130
4.6   US Artefacts   134

Chapter 5   MR Imaging

5.1   MR Machine   139
5.2   Introduction to MRI   141
5.3   T1 and T2 Signal   144
5.4   Spin Echo Sequence   148
5.5   T1, T2 and PD Weighted Imaging   151
5.6   Spatial Encoding   155
5.7   Slice Selection   157
5.8   Frequency Encoding   160
5.9   Phase Encoding   164
5.10 K-Space   166
5.11 Sequences   168
5.12 Spin Echo Sequences - Detailed   170
5.13 Gradient (Recalled) Echo Sequence   173
5.14 Inversion Recovery Sequences   175
5.15 Diffusion-Weighted Imaging   177
5.16 MR Spectroscopy   182
5.17 MR Angiography   185
5.18 MR Contrast Agents   190
5.19 MR Image Quality   192
5.20 MR Artefacts   196
5.21 MR Safety   202

Chapter 6   Molecular Imaging

6.1   Introduction to Molecular Imaging   211
6.2   Non-Nuclear Molecular Imaging   212
6.3   Production of Radioisotopes   215
6.4   Radiopharmaceuticals   219
6.5   Gamma Camera   225
6.6   Planar Imaging   232
6.7   SPECT Imaging   236
6.8   PET Imaging   240
6.9   NM Image Quality   246

6.10   NM Artefacts   252
6.11   NM Quality Assurance   254

Chapter 7   Radiation Dosimetry,
            Protection and Legislation

7.1   Effects of Radiation   259
7.2   Legislation   264
7.3   Radiation Protection   270
7.4   Dosimetry Badges   273
7.5   Patient Dosimetry   275

Appendix

A.   Basic Science   278
B.   X-Ray Imaging   279
C.   CT Imaging   283
D.   Ultrasound Imaging   285
E.   MR imaging   286
F.   Molecular Imaging   288
G.   Radiation Dosimetry, Protection and
       Legislation   291
H.   Miscellaneous   295

Preface

The essence of radiology is physics. A good understanding of the principles that underlie the imaging modalities, and the legislation that governs our practice, is essential. For UK trainees this knowledge is assessed in the first FRCR physics exam.

These beautiful notes are for those sitting the exam and cover the scope of the Royal College of Radiologists syllabus. Indeed, although aimed at radiology trainees the notes provide an excellent overview for anyone interested in learning about the physics of radiology or just refreshing their knowledge.

The notes were created by Dr Sarah Abdulla during her radiology training at the Norfolk and Norwich University Hospitals NHS Foundation Trust. Whilst revising for the first FRCR physics exam she was frustrated by the lack of comprehensive but concise material in an easy to follow format and so created her own notes gathering information from multiple books, journal papers and browser tabs. She soon realised that, perhaps, others had the same problem and might find these notes useful so decided to make them available to everyone online.

These notes have since been moved to Radiology Cafe, a website by Dr Christopher Clarke giving junior doctors invaluable advice on applying to clinical radiology and supporting radiology registrars in training with revision resources and mock exams.

Our goal has been to make the notes concise but comprehensive with plenty of beautiful diagrams to aid in understanding. The clearly organised nature of the notes makes them ideal for dipping into a specific topic for reference, although if you fancy reading the entire physics syllabus, you can do that too. They have been separated into chapters covering basic science, x-ray imaging, CT imaging, ultrasound imaging, MR imaging, molecular imaging, and, radiation dosimetry, protection and legislation.

The content has gone through strict critique and evaluation by physicists and other specialists as well as the users of the website in order to provide an accurate, understandable and up-to-date resource. And now, after the publication of several ebooks and in response to the many requests from users, the new 3rd edition has been transformed and published in paperback (also available as an ebook) with new updates, illustrations and corrections. Hopefully you'll find them useful in your preparation.

We welcome any questions or feedback so please feel free to get in touch with us via the website www.radiologycafe.com.

Enjoy and good luck with your revision!

Dr Sarah Abdulla

Dr Christopher Clarke

Acknowledgements

I would like to thank everyone who has contributed to these notes, in particular the radiographers and medical physics teams at the Norfolk and Norwich University Hospitals NHS Foundation Trust and the medical physics team at Nottingham University Hospitals NHS Trust. Thanks to all the users of the Radiology Cafe website who provided great feedback and gave me the motivation to continue working and complete these notes, and to Tor for her understanding and patience while I spent many evenings editing images and writing code. Finally, and most importantly, I would like to thank my fantastic colleague, Sarah Abdulla, who wrote these amazing notes and made them available for everyone to use. Her dedication and hard work has ensured these notes are helping not only UK trainees, but people all over the world.

- Dr Christopher Clarke

I would first like to thank the Norwich Radiology Academy who allowed me to enter into the world of radiology and supported me throughout my training. I would like to also thank Christopher Clarke for seeing the potential of my primitive online notes and working so hard to create this amazing online and ebook resource. Many thanks to my parents, Anaam and Hassan, who made me believe I could achieve anything and to my siblings, Adam and Tayseer, for keeping my life interesting. And, finally, a grateful thank you to all the users of the notes and their invaluable feedback and comments.

- Dr Sarah Abdulla

We would both like to give a special thanks to Matthew Dunn, Andy Rodgers and Paul Morgan (Medical Physics & Clinical Engineering department at Nottingham University Hospitals), and Mandy Price (Barts Health NHS Trust) for their invaluable help and advice in checking and suggesting numerous amendments to these notes. Thanks also to Melanie Gee who did a fantastic job indexing this text. We are both very grateful.

- Dr Sarah Abdulla & Dr Christopher Clarke

x

1

A knowledge of basic physics is essential to understanding how radiation originates and behaves.

This chapter works through what an atom is; what keeps it stable instead of radioactive and unstable; and if it is unstable, how radioactivity is released.

1.1	Atomic Structure	3
1.2	Electromagnetic Radiation	6
1.3	Radioactive Decay	10

1.1 Atomic Structure

The Rutherford-Bohr Model of An Atom

1) Overview

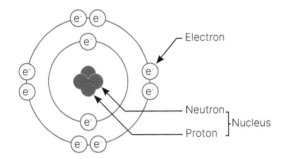

Figure 1   An atom

Atoms consist of:

- **Nucleus**: contains positive protons (p) and neutral neutrons (n)
- **Electrons**: circle the nucleus within energy "shells"

2) Describing an atom

Atoms are displayed in the format shown where:

A = mass number (p + n)
Z = atomic number (protons)
X = chemical symbol of the atom

The neutrons and protons (collectively called **nucleons**) give the atom its mass. This isn't the actual mass but that relative to other atoms.

1 atomic mass unit (amu) = 1/12 the mass of a carbon-12 atom

The amu of different components of the atoms are shown in the table below:

	Relative mass	Charge	Symbol
Neutron	1	0	n
Proton	1	+1	p
Electron	0.0005	-1	e-

Electrons

1) Electron shells

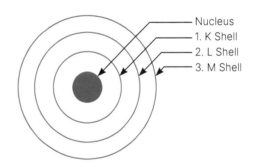

Figure 2   The maximum number of electrons a shell can hold is $2n^2$

The number of electron shells orbiting the nucleus is different depending upon the number of electrons in the atom. A very simplistic model is that each shell has a letter symbol and a maximum number of electrons it can hold calculated by $2n^2$ where n = shell number.

Shell number	Letter symbol	Maximum number of electrons
1	K	$2 \times 1^2 = 2$
2	L	$2 \times 2^2 = 8$
3	M	$2 \times 3^2 = 18$

2) Types of electrons

Electrons are either bound or free.

Bound electrons: These are the electrons that are held in orbit around the nucleus in the electron shells by the attractive force of the positive nucleus. The **binding energy** is the positive energy required to overcome the pull of the nucleus and release the electron from the shell. This is of the same magnitude as the actual (negative) energy of the electron that is released if the electron is freed.

Free electrons: These are the electrons that are not bound in an electron shell around a nucleus. They have a kinetic energy of:

$$\text{Kinetic energy} = \tfrac{1}{2}mv^2$$

Where:
m   =   mass
v   =   velocity

The actual binding energy of electrons is expressed in electron volts (eV) or keV (1keV = 1000 eV)

$$1 \text{ eV} = 1.6022 \times 10^{-19} \text{ joules}$$

3) Key points

- Increase in the atomic number = increase in the binding energy of the electrons (there are more protons and, therefore, more energy is needed to release the electrons from the greater positive pull).
- Increase in the distance between the nucleus and the electron = decrease in the binding energy of the electron (decrease in the positive pull of the protons in the nucleus).

Nuclear Stability

The nucleus is composed of protons and neutrons. The protons repel each other (**electrostatic force**) but the nucleus is kept held together by the **strong nuclear force**.

Strong nuclear force (aka strong interaction): There is a strong force of attraction at distances between nucleons of 1×10^{-15} m (i.e. 1 femtometre, fm) which changes to a repulsive force at $<0.7 \times 10^{-15}$ m. The nucleons are kept apart at a distance of 1 to 2×10^{-15} m, the distance at which there is the greatest attraction.

Electrostatic force (aka coulomb force): this is the force of repulsion between protons. At distances of 10^{-15} to 10^{-16} m the strong attractive interaction (strong nuclear force) is much greater than the repulsive electrostatic force and the nucleus is held together.

4) Segrè chart

The Segrè Chart

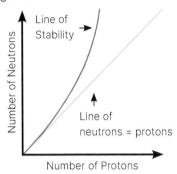

Figure 3   The Segré chart shows the proportion of neutrons needed to keep the nucleus stable as the number of protons increases (the "line of stability")

As the atomic number increases (i.e. the number of protons) more neutrons are required to prevent the electrostatic forces pushing the protons apart and to keep the nucleus stable.

If an atom has too many or too few neutrons and does not lie upon the "line of stability", it becomes unstable and decays to a more stable form. This is the basis of radioactivity and is discussed next in the "electromagnetic radiation" chapter.

- A proton has a mass of 1 and a charge of +1
- An electron has a mass of 0.0005 and a charge of -1
- The mass number (A) of an atom is the number of protons and neutrons
- The atomic number (Z) is the number of protons
- Electrons are held in electron shells that each hold a maximum number of electrons
  - Max no. electrons per shell = $2n^2$, where n = shell number
- Electrons have a binding energy that is the same as their actual negative energy.
  - Binding energy = the positive energy required to release the electron from its shell = the negative energy released by electron when it is freed
- The farther away from the nucleus the electron is the smaller its binding energy
- The higher the atomic number, the greater the binding energy

Summary

- An atom is composed of neutrons, protons and electrons
- Neutrons and protons form the nucleus and, collectively, are called nucleons
- A neutron has a mass of 1 and a charge of 0

1.2   Electromagnetic Radiation

Electromagnetic (EM) radiation arises from oscillating **electric** and **magnetic** fields. It can be considered either as a stream of quanta (photons, particles) or waves.

1) EM radiation as waves

Concerning the wave aspect, it is a sinusoidally varying electric and magnetic field vector with the peaks pointing at right angles to one another and perpendicular to the direction the wave is travelling.

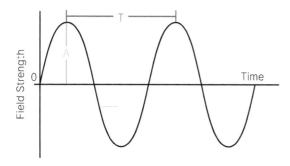

Figure 4   Graph showing wave strength over time

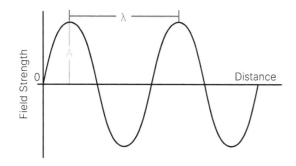

Figure 5   Graph showing wave strength over distance

Definitions

Amplitude (A)	peak field strength	
Wavelength (λ)	distance between successive peaks	Units = m (metres)
Time (T)	time between successive peaks	Units = seconds
Frequency (f)	the number of peaks passing a given point in one second	$f = 1/T$ Units = s^{-1} (per second) or Hz (hertz, 1Hz = 1 cycle per second)
Velocity (c)	the speed calculated as the distance travelled by a peak in one second	$v = f \times \lambda$ (velocity = frequency x wavelength)

2) EM radiation as particles

When considering EM radiation as particles, the particles are small packets, or quanta, of energy called photons that travel in straight lines. The energy of the photon packet is measured in joules (J) but this is inconveniently small when describing EM radiation so the unit of electron-volt is used.

$$1 \text{ ev} = 1.6 \times 10^{-19} \text{J}$$

Intensity

The intensity (i.e. photon energy or field strength) is related to the characteristics of the wave by **Planck's constant**.

$$E = hf$$

Key: E = photon energy
      h = Planck's constant (6.63 × 10⁻³⁴
           m²kg/s)
      f = frequency

Rearranging the earlier equation of velocity = fλ and assuming that the velocity is fixed (i.e. 1) gives you:

$$f = 1 / \lambda$$

In other words, the frequency is inversely proportional to the wavelength. Substituting this into the Planck's constant equation gives you:

$$E = h / \lambda$$

i.e. the photon energy is inversely proportional to the wavelength.

3) Key points

- As the frequency increases, so does the energy of the wave (directly proportional)
- As the wavelength increases the energy of the wave decreases (inversely proportional)

4) Definitions

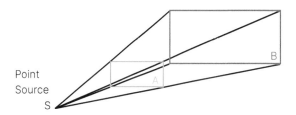

Figure 6   The diagram represents a beam emanating from a point source (S). As the beam moves further from the source it spreads (area B is larger than area A)

Photon fluence = number of photons per unit area at a given time and given cross-section of beam (e.g. number of photons in area A or B).

Energy fluence = total amount of energy of photons at a given time at a given cross-section of the beam per unit area (total energy of photons in area A or B).

Energy fluence rate (aka beam intensity) = total energy per unit area passing through a cross section per unit time (watts/mm²) (total energy per second of photons in area A or B).

5) Inverse square law

As the beam moves further from the source the area of the beam increases. The area of the beam is equal to the distance squared.

$$A \propto d^2$$

Key: A = area
      d = distance

This means the same number of photons are spread over a larger area and the strength of the beam decreases (the intensity is inversely proportional to the area).

$$intensity \propto 1 / A$$

Putting the two equations together gives:

$$intensity \propto 1 / d^2$$

This relationship between the distance from the source and the energy of the beam is called the **inverse square law** as the intensity is inversely proportional to the distance from the source squared.

However, this law only strictly applies if:
▪ Beam comes from point source
▪ No scatter or absorption of the beam

Electromagnetic Spectrum

	Extremely low frequency	Radio waves	Micro-waves	Infrared	Visible light	Ultraviolet	X-rays	Gamma rays
Source	Power line	AM and FM radios	Microwave oven	Radiant heat	Sun	Arc wielding	X-ray tubes	Radio-active sources
Wavelength	km	cm-km	mm-m	microns-mm	400-700 nm	10-400 nm	100-10^{-3} nm	100-<10^{-3} nm
Frequency	30-300 Hz	20 Hz-30 MHz	300 MHz - 300 GHz	300 GHz - 300 THz	430-750 THz	750-3000 THz	3000 THz - 10^{20} Hz	3000 THz to >10^{20} Hz
Photon energy	Pico eV (10^{-12} eV)	Nano to micro eV	Micro to Milli eV	Milli eV to eV	1.8-3.3 eV	3-12 eV	KeV - MeV	KeV - >MeV

Summary

- Radiation is both a wave and particle
- An electromagnetic wave is sinusoidal perpendicular to time and distance
- Frequency = 1 / period (units = s^{-1} or Hz (1 Hz = 1 cycle per second))
- Velocity = f x λ, where f = frequency and λ = wavelength
- Intensity is proportional to frequency
- Intensity is inversely proportional to wavelength
- Inverse square law: intensity inversely proportional to $distance^2$ but only if:
  - Beam comes from a point source
  - No scatter or absorption of the beam

1.3   Radioactive Decay

Radioactive decay generally involves the emission of a charged particle or the capture of an electron by the nucleus to form stable nuclides. The amount of decay = the radioactivity = the number of nuclear transformations per second.

Nomenclature

Nuclide	nuclear species with specific number of neutrons and protons that exists in a defined nuclear energy state (e.g. 99mTc is a different nuclide to 99Tc)
Radionuclide	radioactive nuclide
Metastable radionuclide	a radionuclide that exists for a long time in a higher energy state before falling to ground state (e.g. 99mTc)
Isomer	the <u>m</u>etastable version of a nuclide (iso<u>m</u>er) of a nuclide e.g. 99mTc is an isomer of 99Tc
Isotone	nuclides with the same number of <u>n</u>eutrons (isoto<u>n</u>e) but with a different number of protons
Isotope	nuclides with the same number of <u>p</u>rotons (isoto<u>p</u>e) but with a different number of neutrons

N.B. it is the number of **protons** that determines the **element** of an atom. You can change the number of neutrons (and, therefore, the mass number) and the atom will still be the same element.

Nuclear stability

The line of stability - Segré chart

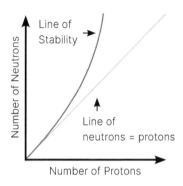

Figure 7   The Segré chart shows the proportion of neutrons needed to keep the nucleus stable as the number of protons increases (the "line of stability")

In the chapter on "Atomic structure" we covered nuclear stability and referred to the Segré chart. What the line of stability shows is that as the number of protons increases, the proportion of neutrons needed to keep the nucleus stable increases. When the nuclide doesn't lie on the line of stability it becomes unstable and radioactive.

Decay model of nuclides

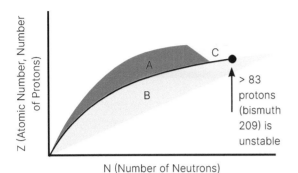

Figure 8   The decay model of nuclides above includes all nuclides; stable and radioactive. Nuclides in area A have too few neutrons, in area B have too few protons, and in area C are very heavy with excess protons and neutrons. The area the nuclide lies in determines the type of radioactivity the nuclide goes through to become stable and is discussed below.

Radioactive Decay

The decay of a nuclide is **exponential** i.e. it theoretically never reaches zero. The S.I. unit of radioactivity is the **Becquerel (Bq):**

1 Bq = 1 transformation per second

1) Types of radiation

When a nuclide undergoes radioactive decay it breaks down to fall into a lower energy state expending the excess energy as **radiation**. The radioactivity released can be in the form of:

1. Alpha particles
2. Beta particles
3. Gamma particles (or photons)
4. Others

1. Alpha particles
- Symbol: α
- Formed of 2 protons and 2 neutrons (i.e. a helium atom)
- Positively charged
- Relatively heavy
- Short range of travel

2. Beta particles
- Symbol: β
- Electrons emitted from radioactive nuclei
- Carry negative charge
- Split into β⁻ (negatron) and an antimatter equivalent β⁺ (positron)
- Lighter and smaller than α

3. Gamma particles
- Symbol: γ
- Identical to x-rays except for the origin (x-rays originate from electron bombardment, gamma particles from radioactive atoms)
- Result of transition between nuclear energy levels
- Very high energy and range of travel

4. Others
- **X-rays**
- **Internal conversion:** γ ray energy transferred to inner shell electron which is then emitted from the nucleus
- **Auger electron:** ejected from electron shells as a result of same radioactive de-

cay processes that create electron shell vacancies. Competes with emission of x-rays.

- **Neutrinos and anti-neutrinos:** electrically neutral particles with very little mass emitted from atomic nuclei during β+ and β- decay respectively.
- **Spontaneous fission:** very heavy nuclides are so unstable they split into two smaller nuclides emitting neutrons in the process.

2) Decay models

There are several ways in which a nuclide can decay to its more stable form. These are:

1. Alpha decay
2. β- decay
3. β+ decay (aka positron emission)
4. Electron capture
5. Isomeric transition
6. Gamma decay

Alpha (α) decay

This occurs in heavier nuclides with too many nucleons. The parent nuclide emits a helium atom (α particle). This type of decay occurs in the nuclides in area **C** of the decay model graph that are very heavy.

$$_{Z}^{A}\text{Parent} \longrightarrow {_{Z-2}^{A-4}}\text{Daughter} + {_{2}^{4}}\text{He}$$

Beta minus (β-) decay

This occurs in nuclides in area **B** of the decay model graph that have too many neutrons. The neutral neutron (n) decays into a positive proton (p) (which is retained in the nucleus), a negative electron (e-) and an electron anti-neutrino (v-e) (i.e. the charge on both sides of the equation remains the same). A neutron is lost and a proton is gained meaning the mass number (A, number of protons plus neutrons) remains equal but the atomic number (Z, number of protons) increases by 1.

$$n \rightarrow p + e^- + v^-e$$

$$_{Z}^{A}\text{Parent} \longrightarrow {_{Z+1}^{A}}\text{Daughter} + e^- + v^-e$$

Beta plus (β+) decay aka positron emission

This occurs in the nuclides in area **A** of the decay model graph that have too few neutrons. The extra proton decays into a neutron (which is retained in the nucleus), a positron (β+ or e) and an electron neutrino (ve). A neutron is gained and a proton is lost meaning the mass number remains equal but the atomic number decreases by 1. This form of radioactivity, with the production of a positron, is important in PET imaging.

$$p \rightarrow n + β^+/e + ve$$

$$_{Z}^{A}\text{Parent} \longrightarrow {_{Z-1}^{A}}\text{Daughter} + e + ve$$

Electron capture

This competes with β⁺ decay as it also occurs in proton-rich nuclei. If the energy difference between the parent and daughter nuclides is too low for positron emission an inner shell electron is captured by the nucleus converting a proton into a neutron (i.e. positive + negative = neutral). As with β⁺ decay the mass number remains the same but the atomic number decreases by 1.

$$p + e^- \rightarrow n$$

Isomeric transition

A radionuclide in a metastable excited state decays to its ground state by isomeric transition and the number of protons and neutrons remain the same. The energy difference is emitted as γ radiation. The mass number and atomic number remain unchanged.

e.g. Tc-99m → Tc-99 + 140 keV γ rays

Gamma (γ) decay

Gamma decay is released by a hyperexcited nucleus to move to lower energy state **after** β or α decay.

3) Points to help understanding

1. The charge on both sides of the equation must remain the same
2. Simplistically speaking, a neutron is made of a proton and an electron

$$n = p + e$$
$$n = +ve + -ve$$

This means:
- A neutron will decay into a proton and an electron (β⁻ decay)
- A proton and an electron will join to form a neutron (electron capture)

3. Simplistically speaking (again) a proton is made of a neutron and a positron (β⁺) (β⁺ decay)

$$p = n + β^+$$
$$+ve = n + +ve$$

4. The mass (A) always remains the same except for in alpha decay

Summary

- The number of protons in an atom determines its element
- Radionuclides transform into a more stable nuclide by releasing energy in the form of radiation
- Radioactivity is measured in Becquerels (Bq). 1 Bq = 1 transformation / second
- Radiation can be alpha, beta or gamma particles
- What is released and the method of decay depends on the characteristics of the radionuclide

Type of decay	Occurs in ...	Produces	Daughter nuclide
Alpha decay	Heavy nuclei	Helium atom (2p and 2n)	A minus 4 Z minus 2
β- decay	Too many neutrons	$n \rightarrow p + e^- + \bar{v}e$ neutron becomes proton and electron	A equal Z plus 1
β+ decay	Too few neutrons Too many protons	$p \rightarrow n + \beta^+ + ve$ proton becomes neutron and positron (β^+)	A equal Z minus 1
Electron capture	Too few neutrons but not enough energy for β+ decay	$p + e^- \rightarrow n$ electron captured and combines with proton to form neutron	A equal Z minus 1
Isomeric transition	Metastable excited nuclides	γ radiation	A equal Z cqual

2

This chapter focuses on the production of an x-ray beam and the utilisation of that beam to create an image. Screen film radiography is rarely used nowadays and does not feature at all in the exams and so is not included in these notes.

2.1   Production of X-Rays   17
2.2   Interaction with Matter   27
2.3   Digital Radiography   34
2.4   Image Quality   43
2.5   Quality Assurance   53
2.6   Mammography   59
2.7   Fluoroscopy   65

2.1 Production of X-Rays

1) Overview

1. A current is passed through the tungsten filament and heats it up.
2. As it is heated up the increased energy enables electrons to be released from the filament through **thermionic emission**.
3. The electrons are attracted towards the positively charged anode and hit the tungsten target with a maximum energy determined by the tube potential (voltage).
4. As the electrons bombard the target they interact via Bremsstrahlung and characteristic interactions which result in the conversion of energy into heat (99%) and x-ray photons (1%).
5. The x-ray photons are released in a beam with a range of energies (**x-ray spectrum**) out of the window of the tube and form the basis for x-ray image formation.

Equipment

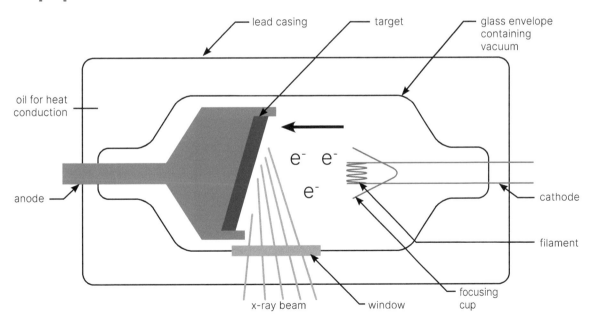

Figure 9   An x-ray tube

2) Cathode

Filament

- Made of thin (0.2 mm) tungsten wire because tungsten:
  - has a high atomic number (A 184, Z 74)
  - is a good thermionic emitter (good at emitting electrons)
  - can be manufactured into a thin wire
  - has a very high melting temperature (3422°c)
- The size of the filament relates to the size of the focal spot. Some cathodes have two filaments for broad and fine focusing.

Focusing cup

- Made of molybdenum as:
  - high melting point
  - poor thermionic emitter so electrons aren't released to interfere with electron beam from filament
- Negatively charged to focus the electrons towards the anode and stop spatial spreading

3) Anode

- Target made of tungsten for same reasons as for filament
- Rhenium added to tungsten to prevent cracking of anode at high temperatures and usage
- Set into an anode disk of molybdenum with stem

- Positively charged to attract electrons
- Set at angle to direct x-ray photon beam down towards patient. Usual angle is 5° - 15°

Definitions

- Target, focus, focal point, focal spot: **where electrons hit the anode**
- **Actual focal spot:** physical area of the focal track that is impacted
- **Focal track:** portion of the anode the electrons bombard. On a rotating anode this is a circular path
- **Effective focal spot:** the area of the focal spot that is projected out of a tube

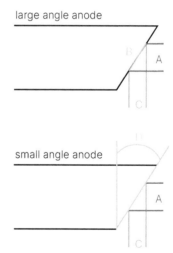

large angle anode

small angle anode

A = bombarding electron beam
B = actual focal spot
C = effective focal spot
D = angle of anode

Figure 10   Anode angles and definitions

Stationary anode: these are generally limited to dental radiology and radiotherapy systems. Consists of an anode fixed in position with the electron beam constantly streaming onto one small area.

Rotating anode: used in most radiography, including mobile sets and fluoroscopy. Consists of a disc with a thin bevelled rim of tungsten around the circumference that rotates at 50 Hz. Because it rotates it overcomes heating by having different areas exposed to the electron stream over time. It consists of:

- Molybdenum disk with thin tungsten target around the circumference
- Molybdenum stem, which is a poor conductor of heat to prevent heat transmission to the metal bearings
- Silver lubricated bearings between the stem and rotor that have no effect on heat transfer but allow very fast rotation at low resistances
- Blackened rotor to ease heat transfer

Heating of the anode

This is the major limitation of x-ray production.

$$\text{Heat (J)} = kVe \times mAs$$
$$\text{or}$$
$$\text{Heat (J)} = w \times kVp \times mAs$$

Key: kVe = effective kV

            w = waveform of the voltage through the x-ray tube. The more uniform the waveform the lower the heat production

            kVp = peak kV

            mAs = current exposure time product

Heat is normally removed from the anode by **radiation** through the vacuum and into the conducting oil outside the glass envelope. The molybdenum stem conducts very little heat to prevent damage to the metal bearings.

Heat capacity

A higher heat capacity means the temperature of the material rises only a small amount with a large increase in heat input.

$$\text{Temperature rise} = \text{energy applied} / \text{heat capacity}$$

Tube Rating

Each machine has a different capacity for dissipating heat before damage is caused. The capacity for each focal spot on a machine is given in tube rating graphs provided by the manufacturer. These display the maximum power (kV and mA) that can be used for a given exposure time before the system overloads. The maximum allowable power decreases with:

- Lengthening exposure time
- Decreasing effective focal spot size (heat is spread over a smaller area)
- Larger target angles for a given effective focal spot size (for a given effective focal spot size the actual focal spot track is smaller with larger anode angles. This means the heat is spread over a smaller area and the rate of heat dissipation is reduced)
- Decreasing disk diameter (heat spread over smaller circumference and area)
- Decreasing speed of disk rotation

Other factors to take into consideration are:

- By using a higher mA the maximum kV is reduced and vice versa.
- A very short examination may require a higher power to produce an adequate image. This must be taken into consideration as the tube may not be able to cope with that amount of heat production over such a short period of time.

Anode cooling chart

As well as withstanding high temperatures an anode must be able to release the heat quickly too. This ability is represented in the anode cooling chart. It shows how long it takes for the anode to cool down from its maximum level of heat and is used to prevent damage to the anode by giving sufficient time to cool between exposures.

Anode heel effect

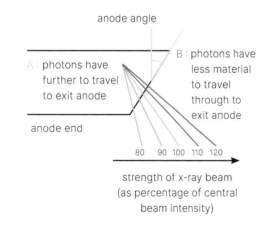

Figure 11   Anode heel effect

An x-ray beam gets attenuated on the way out by the target material itself causing a decrease in intensity gradually from the cathode to anode direction as there is more of the target material to travel through. Therefore, the cathode side should be placed over the area of greatest density as this is the side with the most penetrating beam. Decreasing the anode angle gives a smaller effective focal spot size, which is useful in imaging, but a larger anode heel effect. This results in a less uniform and more attenuated beam.

Smaller angle = smaller focal spot size but larger anode heel effect

4) Others

Window: made of beryllium with aluminium or copper to filter out the soft x-rays. Softer (lower energy) x ray photons contribute to patient dose but not to the image production as they do not have enough energy to pass through the patient to the detector. To reduce this redundant radiation dose to the patient these x-ray photons are removed.

Glass envelope: contains vacuum so that electrons do not collide with anything other than target.

Insulating oil: carries heat produced by the anode away via conduction.

Filter: Total filtration must be >2.5 mm aluminium equivalent (meaning that the material provides the same amount of filtration as a >2.5 mm thickness of aluminium) for a >110 kV generator.

Total filtration = inherent filtration + additional filtration (removable filter)

Producing an X-Ray Beam

1) Electrons produced: thermionic emission

A current is applied through the cathode filament, which heats up and releases electrons via thermionic emission. The electrons are accelerated towards the positive anode by a tube voltage applied across the tube. At the anode, 99% of energy from the electrons is converted into heat and only 1% is converted into x-ray photons.

Accelerating potential

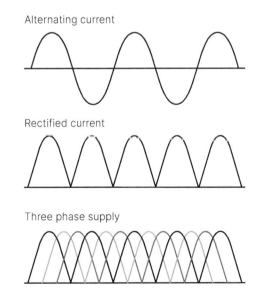

Alternating current

Rectified current

Three phase supply

Figure 12   Accelerating and rectified potentials

The accelerating potential is the voltage applied across the tube to create the negative to positive gradient across the tube and accelerate the electrons across the anode. It is normally 50-150 kV for radiography, 25-40 kV for mammography and 40-110 kV for fluoroscopy. UK mains supply is 230 V and 50 Hz of alternating current. When the charge is negative the accelerating potential is reversed (the cathode becomes positive and the anode becomes negative). This means that the electrons are not accelerated towards the anode to produce an x-ray beam. The ideal waveform for imaging is a positive constant square wave so that the electron flow is continuously towards the anode. We can convert the standard sinusoidal wave into a square wave by rectification.

Full wave rectification: the use of a rectification circuit to convert negative into positive voltage. However, there are still points at which the voltage is zero and most of the time it is less than the maximum kV (kVp). This would lead to a lot of lower energy photons. There are two rectification mechanisms that prevent too many lower energy photons:

Rectification is achieved via two mechanisms:
1. **Three phase supply:** three electrical supplies are used, each applied at a different time. The "ripple" (difference between maximum and minimum current) is about **15%** of the kVp.
2. **High frequency generator:** this can supply an almost constant potential. The sup-

ply is switched on and off rapidly (14kHz) which can then be rectified. They are much more compact than three phase supply and more commonly used.

Effect of rectification on spectrum
- Increased mean photon energy - **fewer photons of lower energy**
- **Increased x-ray output -** stays closer to the maximum for longer
- **Shorter exposure -** as output higher, can run exposure for shorter time to get same output
- **Lower patient dose -** increased mean energy means fewer low energy photons that contribute to patient dose but do not contribute to the final image

Filament current
The current (usually 10 A) heats up the filament to impart enough energy to the electrons to be released i.e. it affects the **number** of electrons released.

Tube current
This is the flow of electrons to the anode and is usually 0.5 - 1000 mA.

Summary
- Filament current is applied across the tungsten cathode filament (10 A) and affects the **number** of electrons released.
- Tube current is applied across the x-ray tube from cathode to anode and affects the **number** of electrons released.

2) X-ray production at the anode

The electrons hit the anode with a maximum kinetic energy of the kVp and interact with the anode by losing energy via:
- **Elastic interaction:** rare, only happens if kVp < 10 eV. Electrons interact but conserve all their energy
- **Inelastic interaction:** causes excitation / ionisation in atoms and releases energy via electromagnetic (EM) radiation and thermal energy

Interactions
At the anode, electrons can interact with the atoms of the anode in several ways to produce x-ray photons.
1. Outer shell interaction: low energy EM released and quickly converted into heat energy
2. Inner shell interaction: produces **characteristic radiation**
3. Nucleus field interaction: aka **Bremsstahlung**

Characteristic radiation

1. A bombarding electron knocks a k-shell or l-shell electron out.
2. A higher shell electron moves into the empty space.
3. This movement to a lower energy state releases energy in the form of an x-ray photon.
4. The bombarding electron continues on its path but is diverted.

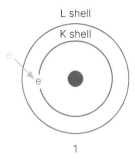

1

Figure 13   Bombarding electron strikes k shell (or other shell) electron.

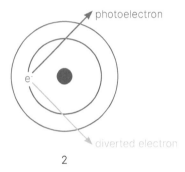

2

Figure 14   Bombarding electron diverted. Electron that's hit ejected as a photoelectron and absorbed.

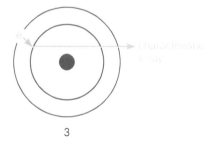

3

Figure 15   Outer shell electron moves down to fill the ejected electron's space. The energy from this is released as a characteristic energy photon.

It is called "characteristic" as energy of emitted electrons is dependent upon the **anode material**, not on the tube **voltage**. Energy is released in characteristic values corresponding to the binding energies of different shells.

For tungsten:

Ek - El (aka Kα) = 59.3 keV

Ek - Em (aka Kβ) = 67.6 keV

Bremsstrahlung radiation

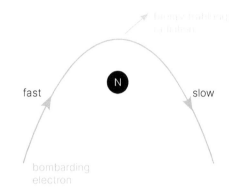

Figure 16   Bremsstrahlung radiation

Bombarding electron approaches the nucleus.

1.   Electron is diverted by the electric field of the nucleus.
2.   The energy loss from this diversion is released as a photon (Bremsstrahlung radiation).

Bremsstrahlung causes a spectrum of photon energies to be released. 80% of x-rays are emitted via Bremsstrahlung. Rarely, the electron is stopped completely and gives up all its energy as a photon. More commonly, a series of interactions happen in which the electron loses energy through several steps.

Characteristic radiation	Bremsstrahlung
Only accounts for small percentage of x-ray photons produced	Accounts for 80% of photons in x-ray beam
Bombarding electron interacts with inner shell electron	Bombarding electron interacts with whole atom
Radiation released due to electron dropping down into lower energy state	Radiation released due to diversion of bombarding electron as a result of the atomic pull
Radiation released is of a specific energy	Radiation released is of a large range of energies
X-ray photon energy depends on element of target atoms not tube voltage	X-ray photon energy depends on tube voltage

Summary of steps

1. **Filament current** applied through tungsten filament at cathode.
2. Heats up filament to produce enough energy to overcome binding energy of electrons (**thermionic emission**).
3. Electrons released from filament.
4. Tube voltage is applied across the x-ray tube.
5. Electrons, therefore, are accelerated towards positively charged anode, which gives them a certain **energy**.
6. The electrons strike the anode and the energy released via interaction with the anode atoms produces **x-ray photons**.
7. These x-ray photons leave the x-ray tube through the window in an x-ray beam towards the patient.
8. They pass through the patient to the detector to produce the x-ray image (this section is covered in the next chapter, 2.2 - Interaction with matter.

X-Ray Spectrum

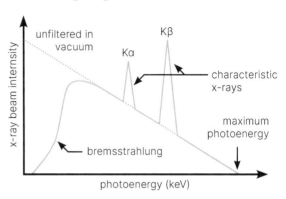

Figure 17   X-ray energy spectrum

The resulting spectrum of x-ray photon energies released is shown in the graph. At a specific photoenergy there are peaks where more x-rays are released. These are at the **characteristic radiation** energies and are different for different materials. The rest of the graph is mainly Bremsstrahlung, in which photons with a range of energies are produced. Bremsstrahlung accounts for the majority of x-ray photon production.

Beam quality: the ability of the beam to penetrate an object or the energy of the beam.

Beam quantity: the number of x-ray photons in the beam

1) Altering the x-ray spectrum

Increasing the Tube Potential (kV)

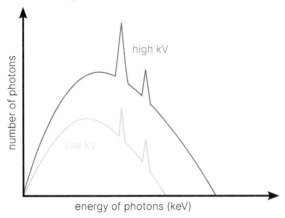

Figure 18   Increasing tube potential

Increased :
- Quantity of x-ray photons
- Average energy
- Maximum energy

If kV great enough, characteristic energy produced

Increasing the Tube Current (mA)

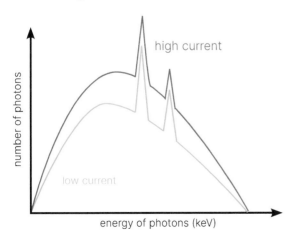

Figure 19   Increasing tube current

Increased quantity of x-ray photons

No change in:
- Characteristic energy
- Average energy
- Minimum energy
- Maximum energy

Filtration

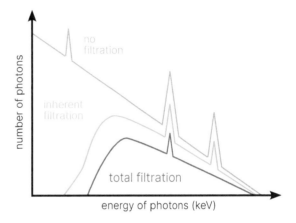

Figure 20   Effect of filtration

Fewer lower energy photons

Increased:
- Average energy of photons

Decreased:
- Total number of photons

Waveform of Current

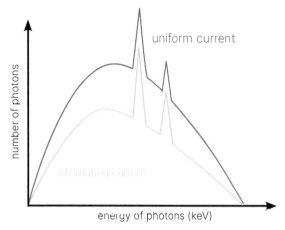

Figure 21   Effect of uniform current

Having a more uniform current (rectified) results in increased:

- Average energy
- Quantity of x-ray photons
- Same maximum keV

Increasing Atomic Number of Target

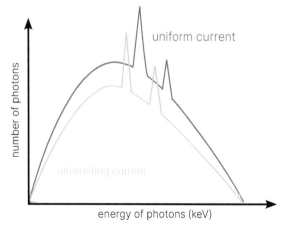

Figure 22   Effect of increasing atomic number of target

Increased:

- Quantity of x-ray photons
- Characteristic energy

2.2 Interaction with Matter

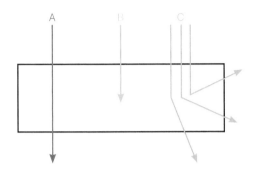

A : transmitted
B : absorbed
C : scattered

Figure 23   Attenuation of X-rays

A beam of x-rays may be:

- **Transmitted:** pass through unaffected or with a lower energy
- **Absorbed:** transfer all energy to matter and not pass through the patient to the film
- **Scattered:** diverted with or without energy loss

Attenuation

Attenuated x-rays are those that are absorbed, transmitted with a lower energy or scattered. It is an exponential process and, therefore, the **beam intensity never reaches zero**. There are two main methods through which attenuation occurs:

- Compton scatter
- Photoelectric effect

Attenuation of the beam can be represented numerically by:

- Half value layer
- Linear attenuation coefficient
- Mass attenuation coefficient

Interactions with matter

Three processes may occur and contribute to attenuation:

- Compton effect (aka Compton scatter, inherent scatter)
- Photoelectric absorption
- Elastic scatter

1) Compton effect

1. X-ray photon hits free/ loosely bound outer shell electron
2. Electron absorbs some of the photon's energy and is deflected
3. The photon, having lost some energy, is deflected and scattered. Because of the production of a scattered photon the Compton effect is considered a scattering process.

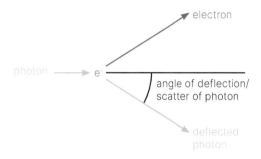

Figure 24 Compton scatter

The Compton effect is also called incoherent scatter as the photon energy change is not always orderly and consistent. The change in energy of the x-ray photon depends on the resulting angle of scatter and not on the scattering medium. The larger the energy discharged by the photon to the electron the:
- Lower the residual deflected photon energy
- Higher the subsequent electron energy
- The larger the angle of the deflected photon

Compton scatter occurs more often with:
- Outer shell electrons
- Loosely bound electrons

Compton attenuating coefficient
This is the probability that an x-ray photon is attenuated via Compton scatter. It is dependent on the number of available electrons; the electron density of the material; and on the physical density but **not on the atomic number of the material**. This is because, with the exception of hydrogen, all materials have approximately the same number of available electrons per gram of material. Materials with a significant proportion of hydrogen have

more electrons per gram and the probability of Compton attenuation is increased.

Compton attenuating coefficient

=

density / energy

Summary
The amount of Compton scatter increases with:
- Increasing mass density
- Increasing electron density of the material
- Lower x-ray beam energy (minimal change over the diagnostic radiation range)

No effect with:
- Atomic number of material (except for materials with significant proportion of hydrogen)

2) Photoelectric effect

1. An x-ray photon interacts with a bound electron from the inner shell.
2. All of the energy of the photon is transferred to the electron.
3. The electron then has enough energy to be freed as a photoelectron and leaves a 'hole' in the shell.
4. The hole is filled by electrons from outer shells. As these electrons move from a lower energy outer shell to a higher energy inner shell, the electrons release the energy at a characteristic energy (i.e. characteristic radiation).

5. The released electron only travels a short distance and deposits its energy into the surrounding matter. In low Z materials (e.g. tissue and bone) the high energy photon collides with a bound electron. The released photon has very little energy and is absorbed immediately with the ejection of a further, low-energy or **"Auger"** electron and all the energy is said to have been absorbed by the material.

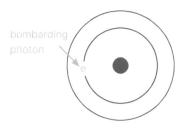

Figure 25   Bombarding photon collides with inner shell

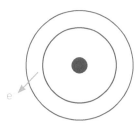

Figure 26   K-shell electron ejected as a photoelectron

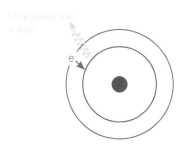

Figure 27   L-shell electron fills k-shell space. The energy released as a photon of characteristic radiation (Ek)

Photoelectric linear attenuation coefficient (LAC)

The probability of photoelectric interactions depends on a few factors as demonstrated in the equation:

- Energy of the x-ray photon
- Atomic number
- Mass density

$$\tau = \rho Z^3 / E^3$$

Key: τ = photoelectric LAC
ρ = mass density
Z = atomic number
E = photon energy

Energy of the x-ray photon

The probability of photoelectric interactions is highest when the x-ray photon energy is slightly above the electron binding energy. If the photon energy is too low it cannot free the electron. If the energy is too high the probability of an interaction significantly decreases due to the inverse relationship with the cube of the energy as demonstrated in the equation for the photoelectric LAC.

As the photon energy increases, there are values where there is a sudden jump in attenuation (k-edge and l-edge). For example, at energies just below the k-edge the photons don't have enough energy to free the k-shell electrons. As the energy increases to just over the required energy, a much larger number of electrons become available for interaction and the probability of the photon being attenuated by a photoelectric reaction significantly increases. This is particularly useful in iodine in which the k-edge is 33 keV, which is in the diagnostic radiation range, and is utilised to massively increase the photoelectric effect and, therefore, give greater tissue contrast.

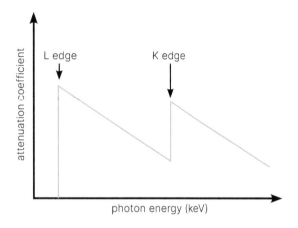

Figure 28   Photoelectric attenuation at increasing energies

Atomic number

An increase in the photoelectric interactions occurs with increasing atomic number as the binding energies of electrons becomes closer to the photon energy.

Summary

The photoelectric effect occurs more often with:

- Inner-shell electrons.
- Tightly bound electrons.
- Incident x-ray energies just higher than the electron-binding energy i.e. closely match the electron-binding energy.

The photoelectric effect increases with:

- Higher atomic number of the material.
- Increasing mass density of the material.

3) Elastic scatter

Aka coherent, classical, unmodified or Rayleigh scattering.

- Photon bounces off an electron that is firmly bound to its parent atom
- Occurs if photon energy less than binding energy of electron
- No secondary electron is set moving and no ionisation or other effect is produced in the material
- Little significance in radiology

4) Competitive interactions

Both photoelectric and Compton scatter contribute to the total attenuation of a beam as it passes through material. The relative contribution of photoelectric and Compton interactions depends on a few factors.

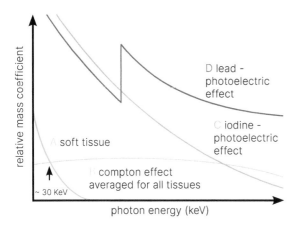

Figure 29   Compton and photoelectric interaction effects on attenuation at increasing photon energies

As the **x-ray photon energy** increases:

▪ There are fewer Compton interactions.

▪ **But** there is a much more significant decrease in photoelectric interactions (i.e. Compton scatter becomes the predominant cause of attenuation at higher energies).

▪ There is a reduction in the total attenuation (i.e. more photons are transmitted through the material).

As the **atomic number** increases:

▪ There is no change in Compton interactions.

▪ Many more photoelectric interactions.

▪ Greater attenuation of the x-ray photons.

As the **tissue mass density** increases:

▪ There is an increase in both Compton and photoelectric interactions.

▪ Greater attenuation of the x-ray photons.

Measuring Attenuation

Half value layer (HVL)

This is the measure of the penetrating power of the **x-ray beam** and is the amount of matter required to attenuate the beam to half its energy value. The smaller the HVL the more attenuating the material is or the weaker the x-ray beam is. It differs for different materials and strengths of beams. To calculate the factor of reduction use: 2^{HVL}

e.g. if the HVL of a beam is 2 mm, by what factor is the beam attenuated if it passes through 8 mm of material?

$$8 \text{ mm} = 4 \text{ HVLs}$$
$$2^4 = 16$$

The beam is attenuated by a factor of 16

Linear attenuation coefficient (LAC)

This is the probability of the **material** to attenuate the beam. It can also be expressed as the amount of energy transferred to the material per unit of track length of the particle. The LAC (μ) is calculated by:

$$\mu = 0.693 / HVL$$

Key: μ = LAC, units: cm^{-1}

Mass attenuation coefficient

The MAC is a measure of the rate of energy loss by a photon beam as it travels through an **area** of material. By dividing LAC by the density of the material the effect of density is removed. The MAC is, therefore, **independent of**

density and depends only on the atomic number of the material and the photon energy.

$$MAC = \mu / \rho$$

Key: μ = LAC, units: cm^{-1}
MAC units : cm^2g^{-1}
ρ = density

5) Effect of beam quality on attenuation

The above only really apply to a monoenergetic (one energy value) beam of x-rays from a point source (infinitely small area) travelling in a vacuum. In reality, the x-ray beam focus is not a fine point and contains photons of different energies that, once they leave the x-ray tube, do not travel in a vacuum.

Wider beam

Increased width of beam = increased scatter produced and measured = larger measured HVL

Heterogeneous beam
- The beams produced by x-ray tubes are photons of a wide range of energies.
- The lower-energy photons are attenuated proportionally more than the higher-energy photons and are removed, leaving behind higher energy photons aka "beam hardening".
- The resulting beam is of a higher average energy.
- It can, therefore, penetrate tissue easier and the HVL is increased.

Summary

- Attenuation is an exponential process - beam intensity never reaches zero
- Penetrating power of a beam is measured by its half value layer (HVL) - the depth of material that results in a 50% reduction in the beam intensity - factor of reduction = 2^{HVL}
- Mass attenuation coefficient independent of density of material - depends only on atomic number of material and photon energy
- Wide beam - increases measured HVL due to increased scatter
- Heterogeneous beam - HVL increases with distance travelled due to beam hardening

Compton effect

Interactions with free / outer shell electrons

Part of photon energy transferred

Depends on:
- Electron density of target
- Physical density of target
- Photon energy (minimally)
- NOT atomic number

More important in low density structures (e.g. air, water, soft tissues) and with high energy photons

Both processes occur equally at:
- 30 keV for air, water and tissue
- 50 keV for aluminium and bone
- 300 keV for iodine and barium
- 500 keV for lead

Photoelectric effect

Interactions with inner shell electrons

Whole of photon energy transferred

Depends on:
- Atomic number of target
- Photon energy
- Physical density of target

More important in high Z structures (e.g. iodine, lead) and with low photon energy

2.3 Digital Radiography

Originally, screen-film radiography (SFR) was used in which a physical copy of the x-ray film was produced. These have now been replaced by digital radiography. There are two different techniques: computed radiography and digital radiography.

Computed radiography

Cassettes are used that have a phosphor screen. When the x-rays hit they form a latent image in the phosphor. The cassette is then placed into a reader with a laser shone on to it which releases the stored photons, collects the signal, and digitises it to be displayed on a display screen.

Digital radiography

With digital radiography no cassettes are used. The x-rays hit a permanently placed set of hardware, which then sends the digital information directly to a readout mechanism.

- **Indirect DR:** x-ray photons hit a **scintillator layer**, which then releases **light photons** that then hit an active matrix array that digitises the signal
- **Direct DR:** x-ray photons act **directly on a photoconductor layer producing positive and negative charge**. The positive charge is attracted to a charge capacitor that stores the latent image. It is then read out by TFT switches pixel by pixel.

Standard DR Process

1. X-ray produced by standard radiographic x-ray tube
2. Image captured by digital image detector
3. Digitised into a stream of data via an analogue-to-digital converter (ADC)
4. Transfer to a system computer
5. Output via digital-to-analogue converter (DAC) to video format
6. Post-processing of image
7. Display on to suitable display device

Computed Radiography (CR)

1) X-ray luminescence

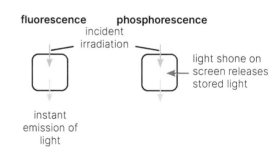

Figure 30 Fluorescence and phosphorescence

X-ray luminescence is the physical mechanism by which x-ray energy is converted into light in a phosphor screen. It involves two mechanisms that both occur to some degree when a phosphor screen is irradiated:

- **X-ray fluorescence:** the immediate emission of light. This is the mechanism that predominates in screen film radiography
- **X-ray phosphorescence:** this is when the emission of light is delayed over a timescale of many minutes, hours or days and can be accelerated by shining specific coloured light onto the phosphor. This is the mechanism exploited in CR. It allows x-ray energy to be temporarily stored in a phosphor screen to be read-out later.

2) CR image plate (CR IP)

The plate is a layer of phosphor crystals (made of barium fluorohalide activated with divalent europium ions (BaFX:Eu)) embedded in a polymer binder with the top surface protected by a layer of toughened plastic. It is typically 0.3 mm thick.

	Standard IP	High resolution IP
Layer of phosphor crystal	Thicker layer	Thinner layer
Crystal size	Larger	Smaller
Light reflection layer	Yes	No
Uses	General radiographic examinations	High spatial resolution
Fractional x-ray absorption efficiency	40% (good)	Lower i.e. need larger x-ray dose

3) Image processing

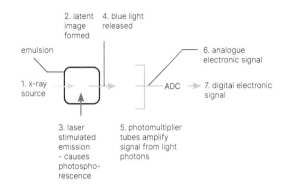

Figure 31   The process of digital radiography

1. Latent image formation
X-ray photons are absorbed into a phosphor crystal giving rise to a high energy photoelectron. This ionises a large number of atoms along its track releasing thousands of electrons (one x-ray photon absorbed gives rise to over 100 trapped electrons). The electrons become temporarily trapped at specific sites throughout the layer of phosphor crystals producing the latent image.

2. Laser simulated emission
If left long enough the electrons spontaneously relax back to their ground state and the image decays over time. During readout the IP is scanned with a **red laser beam** stimulating the trapped electrons to immediately relax back to their ground state and release their stored energy as light photons in the **blue part of the spectrum.** The light photons are then collected by optical fibres to a photomultiplier (PM) tube. The PM tube produces an electrical current.

3. Resetting cassette

Readout is **"destructive"** as it eliminates the latent image. The film is then exposed to bright light to erase any residual signal before re-using the cassette.

4. Post-processing of image

4) Digital image structure

Pixel

Spatial resolution is determined by pixel size. Each pixel records a value, in binary format, related to intensity of signal in the corresponding part of the image. In binary system 1 bit is one value of grey.

N bits = 2^n (number of different values of grey)

Computer memory is measured in bytes:

$$1 \text{ byte} = 8 \text{ bits} (2^8 = 256 \text{ values})$$

5) Image quality

Exposure Index (speed)

The Exposure Index (EI) is a measure of the amount of exposure on the image receptor. In screen-film radiography it is clear if the image is under- or overexposed as it will be too bright or too dark. In computed or digital radiography the image brightness is altered digitally and there is no longer a clear visual link. However, if an image is under or overexposed

this can still affect the image quality by introducing noise or reducing contrast. Manufacturers measure how ideal the exposure is with the EI. Each manufacturer provides a recommended EI range for optimal quality. Each manufacturer has a slightly different method of measuring EI. For example, one manufacturer assesses EI by calculating a "sensitivity number (S-number)" which is calculated as:

$$S - 2000 / X$$

Where:

X = dose incident on the image plate

The S-number usually operates from 200-300.

- S < 200 improved signal to noise ratio but increased patient dose
- S > 400 used when minimal radiation required e.g. repeated paediatric films

Latitude (dynamic range)

Unlike SFR (which has a characteristic curve), the dynamic range is very high and the dose response is linear meaning CR produces good contrast over a much wider range of exposures.

Spatial resolution

Improved by:

- Smaller diameter of readout laser beam (thinner line of image plate "read out")
- Smaller pixels
- Smaller size of phosphor crystals
- Thinner phosphor layer

- No light reflection / absorption backing layer (as this produces scatter despite improving efficiency by using more of the photons for image production)

Spatial resolution is best described by the **modulation transfer function (MTF)**.

Modulation transfer function

The MTF represents the ratio of output to input modulation. An MTF of 1 means the spatial resolution imaged and displayed are the same. As the spatial frequency increases the MTF decreases until, with the addition of noise, it is impossible to visualise details of higher spatial frequencies - the **"limiting spatial resolution"** - and the MTF is 0 (i.e. no information conveyed).

Detective quantum efficiency (DQE) of CR imaging

This is defined by the follow equation:

$$DQE = SNR^2_{out} / SNR^2_{in}$$

Where:
SNR   – signal to noise ratio

The higher the DQE the more efficiently the detector can record information. A DQE of 0.25 implies that the detector can only exploit ¼ of the incident x-ray photons. For a CR imaging system it is typically:
- 0.25 for a standard IP
- 0.12 for high resolution IP

6) Artefacts

Moiré pattern: when a stationary x-ray anti-scatter grid is used there is interference between the linear structure of the grid and the regular pixel array of the digitised image.
Ghost image: due to carry-over of image content from a previous exposure.
Excessively high / low image density: due to faulty operation of the data auto-ranging software, previously due to incorrect identification of the x-ray collimators.
Excessive digital enhancement: e.g. ringing effects along the edges of high density structures or shadowing within such structures.

Digital Radiography

In CR the film cassette has to be removed from under the patient and fed into a reader to be processed. In digital radiography (DR) the image is produced directly from the image detector and is displayed on the screen.

There are two types:
- **Indirect DR:** x-ray → stored electrons → light photons → readout electronics
- **Direct DR:** x-ray → charge → readout electronics

1) Indirect DR

Hardware

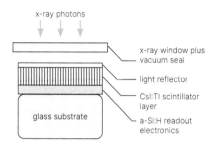

x-ray photons

x-ray window plus vacuum seal

light reflector

CsI:Tl scintillator layer

glass substrate

a-Si:H readout electronics

Figure 32   Digital radiography hardware"

1) Scintillator layer

Most systems use a thin 500 μm layer of **cae-sium iodide (CsI:Tl)** as a scintillator to capture the image which is coated onto the hydrogenated amorphous silicon (a-Si:H) active matrix array (some systems use gadolinium oxysulfide as the scintillator layer). The CsI:Tl is a channeled crystal structure that ensures minimum unsharpness caused by scatter of the recorded image. Absorption of an x-ray photon releases ~3000 light photons in the **green** part of the spectrum.

2) Active matrix

This is formed by a **layer of a-Si:H** and forms the readout electronics. The active matrix consists of a high resolution array of electronic components. Each pixel typically comprises a:

- Photodiode (a light sensor) - amplifies signal from incident light photons
- Charge storage capacitor - stores signal of latent image

- Thin-film transistor (or TFT switch) - latent image read out and transferred to TFT switches that produce a voltage signal that is digitised and converted into the image

This circuitry (TFT and charge storage capacitor) takes up a small area of each pixel preventing image formation in this area. This is calculated by the **fill factor**.

Fill factor = sensitive area / overall area

Decreasing the pixel size (making each area smaller) improves the resolution but, as the circuitry remains the same size, the fill factor and, therefore, the efficiency of the array, decreases.

3) TFT array

This is a device that amplifies the signal then stores it as an electrical charge. The charge can be released and read by applying a high potential. In the array each transistor corresponds to a pixel.

4) X-ray window

The translucent x-ray window is made of aluminium or carbon fibre over the detector entrance to minimise unnecessary absorption and scatter of x-ray photons.

Image formation

1. CsI:Tl absorbs x-ray photons and releases light photons
2. These light photons are then absorbed in

the photodiodes and the charge stored in the charge storage capacitor at each pixel location

3. The latent image is read out sequentially to a bank of charge sensitive amplifier (TFT switches)

4. The resulting voltage signal is then digitised and transferred to the system computer where the DR image is built up

2) Direct DR

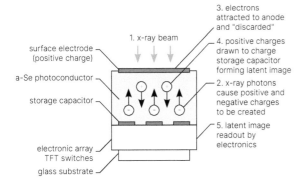

Figure 33   Direct digital radiography equipment

A layer of x-ray photoconductor material is used instead of an x-ray scintillator.

Photoconductor

This directly converts x-ray photon energy into free electrical charge carriers (electrons and holes) i.e. the "middle-men" or light photons, are cut out. The most commonly used photoconductor is **amorphous selenium (a-Se)**.

Sequence of image formation

1. X-ray photon absorbed by a-Se photoconductor

2. Electrical charge carriers (negative electrons and positive holes) are created in the a-Se

3. A surface electrode at positive potential attracts and discards all the electrons

4. The positive charges are drawn to the charge storage capacitor forming the latent image

5. The latent image is then read out sequentially by gating each row of TFT switches (each TFT corresponds to one pixel) in turn to read the charge pattern and transfer to a bank of charge sensitive amplifiers

6. The resulting voltage signal is then digitised and transferred to the system computer where the DR image is built up

7. Post-processing

3) Post-processing

Artefacts and correction

Artefacts

- **Irregular shading across field:** due to non-uniform variations in the sensitivity or gain of the x-ray absorption layer
- **Bright / dark spots or lines in image:** due to individual rows and/or columns of defective pixels in the active matrix array

Correction

- **Gain calibration:** uses previously acquired mask image comprising an image acquired with a uniform x-ray beam and subtracting this gain mask image from the patient's image

- **Pixel-calibration:** defects in pixel array can be corrected by interpolating the data values of neighbouring pixels which are functioning correctly using a reference map

Auto-ranging

The data needs to be matched to the display device.

1. Identification of relevant image field
2. Generation of a histogram of the data representing the number of pixels at each grey-scale value
3. Analysis of the histogram to exclude ranges of data which contain no clinical information (very high and low values)
4. Selected grey-scale range normalised to match the display image

Digital image enhancement

Grey-scale modification

A **look-up-table (LUT)** is a method of systematically re-mapping the grey-scale values in the recorded image to a new range of values in order to improve the displayed image in some way. Shifting the LUT gradient and position adjusts the mean brightness and displayed contrast of the image.

Spatial feature enhancement

1. An unsharp mask algorithm is used to produce a blurred version of the original image
2. This is then subtracted from the original image to produce an image which retains only the fine detail structures in the image

3. Add the fine detail image back onto the original
4. Produces enhanced composite image

Monitor display

Cathode ray tube (CRT)

Visible image generated by scanning a phosphor screen with a focused beam of electrons all contained within an evacuated glass tube.

Flat panel displays

Most display monitors are based on liquid crystal technology. Application of the appropriate voltage distribution to an active matrix modulates light polarisation on a pixel-by-pixel basis varying the light emission that comprises the image seen on the screen. It produces a higher contrast image with greater resolution and less power usage.

Hardcopy

On occasions it is necessary to print a hardcopy image. A hardcopy image is recorded using a laser printer onto a film with silver crystals to create a latent image. This is converted into a visible image by applying heat to the film. This 'dry' film processing eliminates the need for traditional chemical processing.

Summary

1) Computed radiography (CR)

- Image formed on phosphor cassette that is removed, read and then reset to be used again

Process
1. X-ray photons absorbed by phosphor crystal
2. High energy photoelectron released which ionises atoms along its track releasing electrons → >100 electrons released per x-ray photon
3. Cassette removed and placed in machine for read-out
4. Red laser beam scans back and forth releasing energy from electrons, which is released as blue light
5. Light collected by optical fibres to PMT
6. PMT produces electrical current

Image quality
- Exposure Index (speed)
  - Manufacturers calculate a 'sensitivity number (S-number)' to measure this
  - Typically S < 200 → improved SNR but at increased patient dose
  - Typically S > 400 → for when minimal radiation required
- Latitude
  - Dynamic range is a straight line = good contrast over wide range of exposures
- Spatial resolution

- Described by modulation transfer function (MTF): 1 = spatial resolution of image is same as of object. 0 = no information in the image
- Improved by:
  - Smaller readout laser beam
  - Smaller pixels
  - Thinner phosphor layer
  - Smaller phosphor crystals
  - No light reflection / absorption backing layer
- Detective quantum efficiency (DQE)
  - Measure of sensitivity of detector
  - $DQE = SNR^2_{out} / SNR^2_{in}$

2) Digital radiography (DR)

Indirect DR: x-ray photons → light photons → electrical signal
- Process:
  - X-ray photon hits CsI:TI scintillator layer releasing ~3000 green light photons
  - Light photons detected by active matrix of a-Si:H which is separated into pixels with each pixel containing a photodiode and charge storage capacitor
  - Photodiode - amplifies signal
  - Charge storage capacitor - stores signal of latent image
  - TFT switch - latent image read out and transferred to TFT switches that produce voltage signal that is digitised and converted into the image

- Fill factor: TFT and charge storage take up small area of pixel. Fill factor = sensitive area / overall area

Direct DR: x-ray photons → electrical signal
- Process:
  - X-ray photon absorbed by a-Se photoconductor
  - Electrical charge carriers created. The positive charges are drawn to the cathode charge storage capacitor to create latent image
  - Latent image read-out via TFT switches and transferred to bank of charge sensitive amplifiers
  - Voltage signal digitised

Post-processing
- Artefacts:
  - Irregular shading due to non-uniform variation in sensitivity or gain
  - Bright / dark spots due to individual row / column of defective pixels
- Correction of artefacts:
  - Gain-calibration uses mask image obtained with uniform x-ray beam to correct patient image
  - Pixel-calibration uses values of neighbouring pixels to correct defects in pixel array
- Auto-ranging:
  - Analysis of histogram of image grey-scale data to reject very high and low values that contain no clinical information

- Digital image enhancement:
  - Grey-scale modification - look-up-table (LUT) to remap grey-scale values and improve displayed image
  - Spatial feature enhancement to produce enhanced composite image

2.4   Image Quality

There are certain qualities of an image that affect each other and determine the quality of the displayed image:

1. Contrast
2. Resolution
3. Noise

As well as:

4. Unsharpness
5. Magnification
6. Distortion
7. Artefacts

Contrast

Contrast is the difference in the displayed or image signal intensity between two areas of interest e.g. a lesion and background tissue. A high contrast image has a greater difference between the grey shades displayed but a smaller range of greys. A low contrast image has a smaller difference (i.e. it's more difficult to make out different areas) but a larger range of greys.

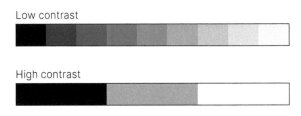

Low contrast

High contrast

Figure 34   High and low contrast

1) Subject contrast

Subject contrast is the ratio of the radiation intensities in different parts of an image due to the quality of the **subject** being imaged. The contrast is due to the differential attenuation by the tissues.

$$c \propto (\mu_1 - \mu_2) \times t$$

Where: c = contrast

μ = attenuation coefficient of object 1 and 2 in the material being imaged

t = thickness of the structure

From the above equation you can see that a higher contrast is achieved with:

- Thicker structure being imaged
- Greater difference between the attenuation of the two objects

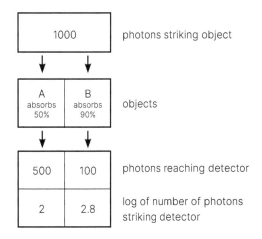

Figure 35   Subject contrast

In the diagram (Fig 35) tissue A absorbs 50% of the radiation incident upon it, B absorbs 90%. If there are 1000 photons for every element of the image then 500 photons will emerge from A and 100 from B (a ratio of 5:1).

As optical densities (the displayed shade in the image) vary with the log of the exposure log500 = 2.7 and log100 = 2.0 so the subject contrast has a difference in the logs of 0.7.

Factors affecting contrast

Linear attenuation coefficient of subject

The linear attenuation coefficient depends on the Compton and the photoelectric linear attenuation coefficient (LAC).

$$Compton\ LAC = \rho / E$$
$$Photoelectric\ LAC = \rho Z^3 / E^3$$

Where: ρ = density
E = energy (kV)
Z = atomic number of material

From the equations above we can see contrast can be improved by:
- Decreasing the energy (tube potential kV)
- Increasing the difference in Z (atomic number) (e.g. use of iodine or barium as a contrast medium against soft tissue)
- Increasing the difference in ρ (density) (e.g. use of barium or gas as a contrast medium)

Overlying tissue

If there is overlying tissue over both A and B, subject contrast is not changed as the same ratio of photons is still absorbed in tissues A and B.

Scatter

Suppose scatter contributes an additional 50 photons to each element in the image. There will now be 550 photons in the film under tissue A and 150 under tissue B. The ratio of signals is now 3.6 (550/150) and the difference in logs is 0.6 (was 0.7) i.e. a reduced contrast.

Scatter is reduced by:
- Using an anti-scatter grid
- Using a larger air gap

Summary

Improved contrast
- Thicker structure
- Greater attenuation between objects
- Decreasing kV
- Increasing difference in Z of objects
- Increasing difference in density of objects

Reduced contrast
- Increased scatter

No effect
- Overlying tissue

2) Image contrast

Image contrast, or radiographic contrast, is the difference in density between neighbouring regions on the image.

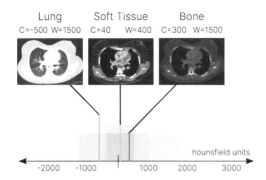

Figure 36 Digital windowing

Image contrast is altered by windowing on the viewing monitor. Images are presented at a certain **width** and **centre** of Hounsfield units displayed. The larger the width, the larger the range of shades displayed and, therefore, the smaller the difference in contrast between each shade. The window is adjusted for the Hounsfield unit of the tissues that need to be assessed.

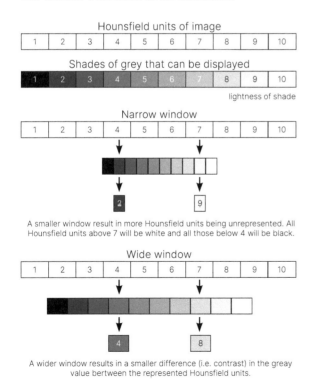

Figure 37 Explanation of windowing

Spatial Resolution

Resolution is the measure of how far apart two objects must be before they can be seen as separate details in the image. There are several ways to measure spatial resolution.

1) Measuring spatial resolution

Line spread function

This is a measure of how spread out the image of a sharp object becomes. However, this is difficult to calculate and it is easier to look at the image in terms of spatial frequency content.

Spatial frequency

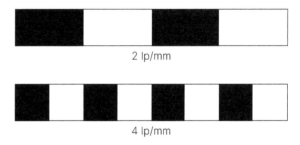

Figure 38 Spatial frequency in line pairs per mm

This is measured in **line pairs per mm (lp/mm)**. An image with a high lp/mm is a high spatial frequency image as there are many alternating light and dark regions in a single millimetre. We, therefore, need a system that can reproduce the image with the appropriate frequency. The lp/mm of different radiographic techniques can be found in the appendix.

How well a system is able to represent the object spatial frequency is expressed as the **modulation transfer function (MTF)**.

Modulation transfer function

MTF = 1   Same range is obtained in the image

MTF < 1   Lower range in the image

MTF = 0   No information in the image

E.g for an imaging system that can fully change from black to white over 1 mm:
For images with 0.5 lp/mm, it gives an MTF of 1
For images with > 0.5 lp/mm, it gives an MTF of <1

MTF is calculated from the line spread function using Fourier transform analysis. The total MTF is the product of the MTF of all constituent parts of the imaging system.

Factors affecting spatial resolution

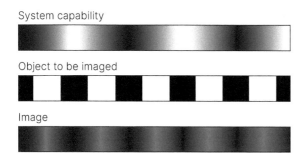

System capability

Object to be imaged

Image

Figure 39   System spatial resolution

- If the **object spatial frequency** is too high for the system, the system will be unable to display the image adequately. The higher the object spatial frequency, the lower the MTF until the system cannot distinguish the line pairs at all resulting in a homogeneous grey i.e. MTF = 0.
- If the object has **low contrast** the system will reach an MTF of 0 earlier as the smaller difference in the range of shades means that the image will reach a homogeneous grey much sooner than if it was a high contrast image (e.g. alternating bands of black and white).
- Anything that increases the **unsharpness** will blur the edges and further reduce the spatial frequency.

2) Digital detectors

There are several things that affect the resolution of digital detectors.

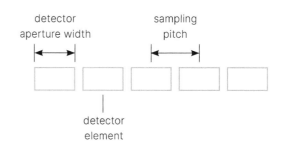

Figure 40   Detector properties

Detector aperture

This signal is averaged over the area of the detector element. If object details are much smaller than the size of the element they are not visible unless they have enough contrast to have a significant effect on the average signal.

Sampling pitch

This is the centre-to-centre distance between individual detector elements. It determines the highest spatial frequency that can be imaged: the **Nyquist frequency**.

Nyquist criterion states that the sampling frequency must be at least twice the highest signal frequency. The highest signal frequency is also called the **"Nyquist frequency"** i.e. for a system to be able to accurately represent the spatial resolution of the object it must have the appropriate sampling pitch which is no less than double the object spatial frequency.

Sampling frequency = 2 x Nyquist frequency

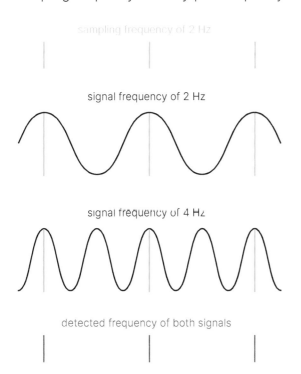

sampling frequency of 2 Hz

signal frequency of 2 Hz

signal frequency of 4 Hz

detected frequency of both signals

Figure 41   Sampling frequency limit

Noise

There is random variation in the number of photons forming each part of the image, called **noise**, that can obscure the signal received from the subject. The amount of quantum noise produced increases with an increasing total number of photons. We usually express this random variation as the standard deviation which is best estimated by the square root of the average number of photons per area.

$$\text{Quantum noise} \propto \sqrt{\text{photons}}$$

However, when we calculate the quantum noise as a proportion of the total signal we can see that the **proportion** of noise in the signal actually decreases with an increasing photon concentration.

$$\text{Noise} \propto 1 / \sqrt{\text{photons}}$$

Average number of photons absorbed by each detector (N)	1000	100
Noise	$\sqrt{1000} = 31.6$	$\sqrt{100} = 10$
Proportion of signal which is noise	$31/1000 \times 100 = 3\%$	$10/100 \times 100 = 10\%$
Signal to noise ratio (SNR) = N / $\sqrt{N}$	31	10

Reducing the proportion of noise in an image will improve the quality. The main way to achieve this is to increase the number of photons detected and used to form each image pixel / element. This can be done in several ways.

- Increasing the **dose (mA):** higher number of photons and smaller proportion of noise
- Using an image receptor with a **greater attenuation coefficient**: more photons are absorbed and converted into a signal
- Make the image receptor **thicker:** again, more photons will be absorbed and converted into a signal
- Using **larger detector elements:** more area to absorb photons per pixel. However, the spatial resolution will decrease

Factors that don't reduce noise
- **Amplification:** attaining a higher signal from each absorbed photon, either by using a faster film-screen combination or gain of an image intensifier would just amplify the signal from noise as well
- Using a narrower window to produce a **high contrast image**

Unsharpness

There are four causes of unsharpness:
- Geometric unsharpness
- Image receptor unsharpness
- Movement unsharpness
- Edge unsharpness

1) Geometric unsharpness

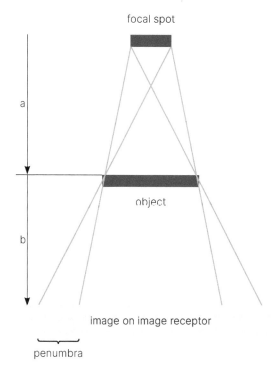

Figure 42   Geometric unsharpness

The boundaries between a dark and a light area may be ill-defined, resulting in a blurred edge. This is called **"unsharpness"**. There are several causes and types of unsharpness as outlined below.

The focal spot is not infinitely small. There will be areas of the image that are:
- High signal: all x-ray photons reach detector
- Low signal: no x-ray photons have passed through the object to reach the detector
- Intermediate: not all photons have passed through the object. The size of this area determines the unsharpness and is called the **penumbra**.

Moving an object closer to the focal spot will increase the penumbra and, therefore, the unsharpness.

The geometric unsharpness (U_g) is determined as follows:

$$U_g = f \times b / a$$

Where:
f   = x-ray focal spot size
a   = distance from x-ray source to front surface of object
b   = distance from object to detector

2) Image receptor unsharpness

- **Digital images:** if a detector element lies across the border between a light and a dark area the pixel displayed will be an average of these two values creating a blurred border.

3) Movement unsharpness

If an object moves during the acquisition the edge will be blurred resulting in unsharpness.

4) Edge unsharpness

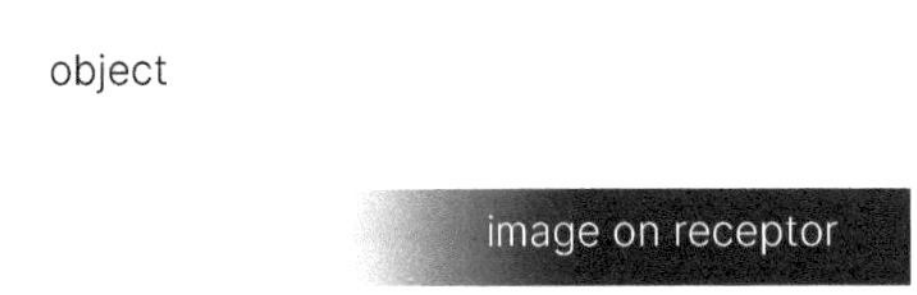

object

image on receptor

Figure 43   Edge unsharpness

If an object has a tapering edge the attenuation will gradually decrease along the object.

Magnification

Magnification (M) depends on the relative distance of the object between the x-ray source (focal spot) and the image receptor. The further from the detector the object is the more the image is magnified.

$$M = \text{image size} / \text{object size}$$
$$= d2 / d1$$

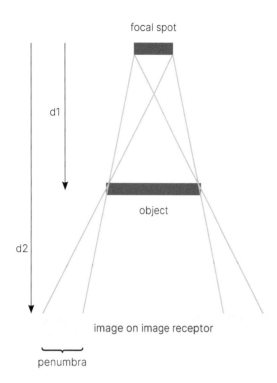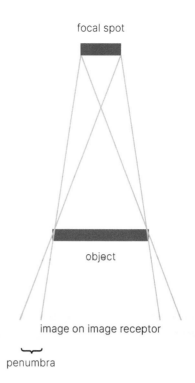

Figure 44   Magnification artefact

Distortion

Depending on the angle at which the x-ray beam passes through an object it can distort the shape and create a distortion artefact.

Artefacts

There are a variety of patient and system factors that can create artefacts:

- Motion artefact
- Double exposure
- Grid cut off
- Radio-opaque objects on or external to the patient

Summary

1) Contrast

- Difference in attenuation (subject contrast) or displayed shade (image contrast) of an image

Subject contrast

- contrast proportional to $(\mu_1 - \mu_2) \times t$ - where: μ = attenuation coefficient of object 1 and 2, t = object thickness
- Improve contrast by:
  - Thicker object
  - Greater attenuation between objects
  - Decreasing kV
  - Increasing Z (atomic number) differ-

ence in objects
- Increasing difference in density of objects
- Contrast reduced by:
  - Increased scatter (no anti-scatter grid, smaller air-gap used)
- No effect:
  - Overlying tissue

Image contrast
- Digital imaging system: achieved by windowing at the imaging monitor

2) Spatial resolution

- Measure of how far apart two objects must be before they can be seen as separate details in an image

Measured as:
- Line spread function: how spread an image of a sharp object becomes. Difficult to measure
- Line pairs per mm (lp/mm)

Accuracy of system display of object spatial frequency = **modulation transfer function (MTF)**
- MTF = 1 same range obtained
- MTF < 1 smaller ranger obtained
- MTF = 0 no information in image

Factors affecting spatial resolution:
- Object properties:

- Object spatial frequency: if it is too high for the system it will not be displayed accurately
- Object contrast: lower contrast objects reach an MTF of 0 at lower spatial frequencies
- Computed / digital radiography:
  - Detector element size: smaller element = higher spatial resolution
  - Distance between detector elements: smaller distance = higher spatial resolution
- Others:
  - Anything that increases unsharpness

3) Noise

- Noise inversely proportional to √photons
- Reducing noise: anything that increases number of x-ray photons (x-ray beam) produced and absorbed and the number of light photons (at the image receptor) produced:
  - Increasing dose (mA)
  - Using an image receptor with a greater attenuation coefficient
  - Making the image receptor thicker
  - Using larger detector elements

Factors that don't reduce noise:
- Amplification
- Using narrower window to produce a high contrast image

Unsharpness

- Geometric unsharpness
  - Focal spot not infinitely small, therefore, blurred penumbra produced at object edge
  - $U_g = f \times b / a$ - where f = x-ray focal spot size, a = distance from focal spot to object, b = distance from object to detector
- Image receptor unsharpness
  - Digital images: if detector element straddles light and dark area pixel displayed will be an average of these two values
- Movement unsharpness
- Edge unsharpness

Magnification

- Greater magnification by moving object further from detector and closer to x-ray tube

Distortion

- Due to the finite size of the focal spot an image may be distorted depending on the angle at which it is imaged

Artefacts

- These may be due to patient or system factors

Speed

- Speed = 2000 / x where x = dose incident on IP
- S < 200 = improved SNR but increased patient doses

Spatial resolution

- Measured by MTF
- Detective quantum efficiency (DQE) = SNR^2_{out}/SNR^2_{in}
  - Greater DQE = more efficient detection of incident x-ray photons
- Improved by:
  - Smaller diameter of readout laser beam
  - Smaller pixels
  - Smaller size of phosphor crystals
  - Thinner phosphor layer
  - No light reflection / absorption backing layer (produces scatter)

2.5 Quality Assurance

Quality assurance is a requirement of IRR 2017 and each hospital should establish its own **quality manual** detailing:
- What tests have to be done
- How the tests should be done
- How often the tests should be done
- How the test results are recorded and analysed
- What the acceptable margin of deviation from the standard is
  - If test differs by a margin that requires action to rectify it = remedial level
  - If test differs by a substantial margin that means equipment no longer fit to use = suspension level
- What to do if a test is failed

Institute of Physics and Engineering in Medicine (IPEM) report 91: Recommended standards for the routine performance testing of diagnostic x-ray systems.

IPEM report 91 divides QA tests into two levels, which it calls level A and level B.
Level A tests:
- Are generally quick and simple
- Do not need expensive or complex equipment
- Do not need detailed analysis
- Are done frequently
- Are usually done by the equipment user
Level B tests:
- Take longer
- Might require expensive or complex equipment
- Need more analysis
- Might be done less frequently than level A tests
- Are often done by medical physics departments or by manufacturers' engineers

X-Ray Set Tests

1) X-ray tube output

- Test every 1-2 months
- Ionisation chamber placed at a known distance from the x-ray tube. The measurements of dose (using an electrometer) are made for various exposures to determine:
  - Dose per mAs (output) for range of exposures
  - Whether output varies with mA
  - How output varies with kV
  - Repeatability - Whether output is consistent when same exposure repeated
    - Remedial level **= +/- 10%**
    - Suspension level **= +/- 20%**
  - Consistency - whether output has changed since the baseline set of QA checks
    - Remedial level **= +/- 20%**
    - Suspension level **= +/- 50%**

2) X-ray tube kV

- Test every 1-2 years
- Potential measured using an electronic kV meter. The kV is then measured at a range of different exposure settings.
  - Is it accurate - do we get the value we have selected?
  - Does it change if we change the mA range or exposure time?
  - Does it vary during the exposure?
- **Remedial level** = +/- 5% or +/- 5 kV from baseline, whichever is greater.
- **Suspension level** = +/- 10% or +/- 10 kV from baseline.

3) Filtration

- N.B. not regularly measured as doesn't change.
- Dose for fixed exposure measured with varying thicknesses of aluminium placed in the beam.
- The thickness that gives 50% transmission (half original dose) is the half-value thickness (HVT) or half value layer (HVL).
- Data is available that enables the filtration to be estimated from the HVT.

4) Automatic exposure control

- Some tests are done for level A and some for level B.
- The AEC terminates the exposure once the film has received an appropriate level of dose.
- It should produce a consistent optical density in the film for a wide range of tube potential (kV) and for a wide range of patient thickness.
- Perspex or water blocks used to simulate a patient
- A series of exposures at different tube voltages and using a different thickness of material is taken.
- The mAs and the detector dose indicator measurement is recorded.
- AEC sensitivity
  - **Tested** every 1-3 months
  - A 1 mm copper in the beam is imaged with exposure under the AEC device control then the whole detector is irradiated. The mAs and detector dose indicator (DDI) reading is then recorded.
  - **Remedial level** = baseline ± 25%
  - **Suspension level** = baseline ± 50%
- Guard timer operation
  - Tested **annually**
  - The guard timer terminates the exposure after a certain amount of time
  - It is tested by using a low kV exposure with lead blocking the AEC chambers and ensuring the exposure is terminated at the guard timer setting.
- AEC consistency
  - Tested **annually**
  - The DDI and mAs is checked between the AEC chambers to ensure consistency between them.

    Remedial level = baseline ± 30%, mean ± 20%
- AEC repeatability

    Tested **annually**

    The mAs and DDI of successive repeated exposures is measured using the same AEC settings

    Remedial level **= mean ± 20%**
- AEC reproducibility

    Tested **annually**

    Testing is similar to the AEC consistency tests but a larger range of kV and thickness of phantoms is used.

    Remedial level = baseline ± 30%

    Suspension level = baseline ± 60%

5) Light beam alignment

- Tested every **1-2 months**.
- Edges of light beam marked on film and film exposed. Area of exposed field then compared to light field
- **Remedial level** = 1 cm misalignment on any side at 1 m from focal spot
- Suspension level **= 3 cm**

6) Focal spot measurement

N.B. most physics services do not measure this regularly as it doesn't change and any faults can be picked up from the image quality and tube output tests.

Pinhole
- Pinhole a few microns across (smaller than the focal spot) radiographed.
- Taking into account the distance from the focus to the pinhole and the focus to film distance you can then calculate the size of the focal spot by measuring the image produced on the film.
- Can estimate size, shape and irregularities in the focal spot with this method

Star test object
- An array of radiating lead spokes is imaged with a geometric magnification of approximately 3
- The spokes at the centre will come to a point at which they can no longer be distinguished by the system due to being too small and close together.
- The diameter of the blurred area can be used to calculate the focal spot size

CR and DR radiography

There are a few tests specific to computed and digital radiography as outlined below.

1) Detector dose indicator (DDI)

- The detector dose indicator measures the dose received at the detector. There are several tests performed to guarantee the accurate functioning of the DDI.

- DDI repeatability and reproducibility
  - Tested **annually**
  - **Remedial level** = baseline ± 10%
  - **Suspension level** = baseline ± 20%

2) Image quality

- Low contrast sensitivity
  - Tested every **4-6 months**
  - The Leeds Test Objects Ltd is used to ensure the system is still able to image low contrast items
  - **Remedial level** = baseline ± 2 groups
- Threshold contrast detail detectability
  - Measured **annually**
  - A test object with an appropriate filter and kV is imaged and the contrast that can be accurately imaged is measured.
- Limiting spatial resolution
  - Tested every **4-6 months**
  - A lead grating resolution bar pattern is used to assess the highest spatial resolution the system can image accurately
  - **Remedial level** = baseline minus 25%
- Uniformity of resolution
  - Tested **annually**
  - A fine wire mesh is imaged and checked for blurred areas and discontinuities
  - **Remedial level** = increase in blurring from baseline
- Measured uniformity
  - Tested **annually**

- An image is obtained with no object in the field. An ROI is then placed over each quadrant and in the centre. The 5 values are used to calculate the standard deviation divided by the mean value.
- Remedial level **= mean ± 5%**
- Dark noise
  - Tested **annually**
  - An image is obtained without exposure or with very low exposure. This tests for noise in the system.
  - **Remedial level** = baseline ± 50%
- Scaling errors
  - Tested **annually**
  - A grid and an attenuating object of known dimensions or a lead ruler are used to ensure that the scale of the image is correct.
  - **Remedial level** = > 2% difference

Summary

- Quality assurance is a requirement of **IRR 1999** but exact schedule and test list is not specified - up to individual hospital
- **IPEM report 91** provides guidelines
- Remedial level = action required to improve equipment performance
- Suspension level = equipment should not be used anymore. Not every piece of equipment has a suspension level

1) Example testing timeline and summary

Equipment tested	Frequency of testing	Method of testing	Performance criteria
X-ray tube output	1-2 months	Dose at various exposures measured with ionisation chamber at known distance	Repeatability: ▪ Remedial = ± 10% ▪ Suspension = ± 20% Consistency: ▪ Remedial = ± 20% ▪ Suspension = ± 50%
Light beam alignment	1-2 months	Light beam field compared to exposed field on film	Remedial = 1 cm misalignment on any side at 1 m from focal spot Suspension = 3 cm
Automatic exposure control (AEC) sensitivity	1-3 months	1mm copper imaged with exposure under AEC device control. mAs and DDI reading recorded.	Remedial = baseline ± 25% Suspension = baseline ± 50%
Low contrast sensitivity	4-6 months	Uses Leeds Test Object Ltd test object	Remedial = baseline ± 2 groups
DR/CR limiting spatial resolution	4-6 months	Uses lead grating resolution bar pattern	Remedial = baseline minus 25%
AEC ionisation chamber consistency	Annual	Expose ionisation chambers separately and compare (usually three)	Remedial = baseline ± 30%, mean ± 20%
AEC repeatability	Annual	mAs and DDI of successive repeated exposures measured	Remedial level = mean ± 20%
AEC reproducibility	Annual	Similar to AEC consistency but larger range of kV and thickness of phantoms used	Remedial level = baseline ± 30% Suspension level = baseline ± 60%
Focal spot	Annual	**Pinhole** Pinhole radiographed and size, shape and inconsistencies of focal spot calculated from image produced **Star test object** Radiating lead spokes radiographed and central blurred area size used to calculate focal spot size	
Filtration	Annual	Half value thickness / layer of filter determined and compared to available data to calculate filtration Should be equivalent to 2.5 mm aluminium	

Equipment tested	Frequency of testing	Method of testing	Performance criteria
Detector dose indicator repeatability and reproducibility	Annual		Remedial = baseline ± 10% Suspension = baseline ± 20%
Threshold contrast detail detectability	Annual	Test object with appropriate filter and kV imaged	
Uniformity of resolution	Annual	Fine wire mesh imaged	Remedial = increase in blurring from baseline
Scaling errors	Annual	Grid imaged with object of known length	Remedial = >2% deviation from object
Dark noise	Annual	No exposure or low exposure	Remedial = baseline + 50%
Measured uniformity (DR/CR)	Annual	Image obtained with no object. ROI over each quadrant and centre. Mean and standard deviation calculated	Remedial level = mean ± 5%
X-ray tube kV	1-2 years	Electronic kV meter measures kV at different exposure settings	Remedial = ±5% or ±5 kV from baseline Suspension = ± 10% or ± 10kV from baseline

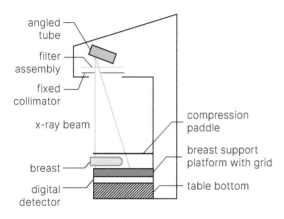

2.6 Mammography

Equipment

angled tube
filter assembly
fixed collimator
x-ray beam
breast
digital detector

compression paddle
breast support platform with grid
table bottom

Figure 45 Mammography machine

Angled Tube Head
Due to the anode heel effect, the x-ray beam is not uniform in the direction parallel to the anode-cathode axis of the x-ray tube. This property is used in mammography by aligning the cathode over the chest wall end (higher energy beam to image thicker area) and the anode over the nipple end (lower energy beam can penetrate thinner area).

C-Arm Design
The x-ray set is a c-arm. The whole gantry rotates so that the tube and breast table remain opposite each other.

Fixed Focus-Detector Distance (FDD)
The set is designed for a single examination and the focus-detector distance (FDD) or focus-to-film distance (FFD) of 65-66cm is considered optimum. This set FDD is a compromise between lower patient doses (lower doses with higher FFDs) and higher film doses (lower exposures with higher FFDs). Also, higher FDDs require longer exposures for a fixed mA resulting in more movement unsharpness.

Compression Device
The maximum force applied should be no greater than 200 N (approx. 20 kg weight). Standard compression forces are normally between 100 - 150 N. The compression plate is angled so that more of the breast is in contact with the compression paddle.

Fixed Field Size
Unlike in general radiography, only one type of examination is done meaning collimation creating fixed field sizes are all that are required.

Grids
Moving anti-scatter grids are used in normal mammography imaging. For magnification views, the breast support table is above the film to give magnification factors of around 1.8. In this case the large air gap between the breast and the film works to reduce scatter and so no grid is needed.

Automatic Exposure Control (AEC)
In screen-film mammography a separate

AEC was required placed behind the cassette. With the currently used digital mammography the detectors act as the AEC. In screen-film radiography an AEC is required to ensure a suitable exposure to prevent under- or over-exposed film. In digital radiography, however, windowing can negate the effects of unsuitably exposed film and the AEC is more to ensure a suitable radiation dose for the patient and for the working parameters of the digital detector.

Target / Filter Material

- Need good differentiation of low contrast structures
- Need very high spatial resolution for micro-calcifications

Target
Need material that produces characteristic x-rays with energies of 17-20 keV (20-30 keV for larger breasts) to produce the best contrast. The commonly used material is Molybdenum (characteristic x-rays at 17.5 and 19.6 keV).

Filter
A filter with a k-edge of an energy just above the characteristic energies is used to remove the higher energy x-ray photons and make the beam as monoenergetic as possible. Molybdenum has a k-edge of 20 keV, just high enough so that the large increase in attenuation (k-edge) doesn't fall into the characteristic energies produced at the molybdenum target.

Alternatives
Mostly MoMo (molybdenum target, molybdenum filter) but this does not give high enough energies for larger breasts.

- **Rhodium** has a k-edge at 23.3 keV and we can use a molybdenum target and rhodium filter (MoRh) to increase the amount of x-rays with energies in the range of 20 - 23.3 keV.
- **Rhodium** characteristic x-rays are at 20.2 - 22.7 keV. When used as a target this produces a beam with a mean energy that is higher than for MoMo and for MoRh.
- **Tungsten** (W) target and **Rhodium** filter. The x-ray output is reduced as no characteristic x-rays are produced (and, therefore, longer exposure times) but tungsten is much cheaper. It is mostly used in breasts with implants or that have been treated with radiotherapy as they are much larger and denser.

	Contrast	Radiation dose
Highest	MoMo	MoMo
	MoRh	MoRh
	RhRh	RhRh
Lowest	WRh	WRh

The mean energy of the spectrum decreases from WRh to MoMo. Lower energy photons have a higher probability of interacting with matter and, therefore, produces better contrast. However, the lower the energy, the greater the absorption, the more energy is deposited in the matter, and the higher the dose.

Summary
- General use: MoMo
- Dense breasts: MoRh or RhRh

Spatial Resolution

A very high resolution is required to see microcalcifications. This is achieved via:
- Focal spot size
- Compression
- Anti-scatter grid

1) Small Focal Spot Sizes

Broad focal spot size = 0.3 mm

Fine focus focal spot size = 0.1 to 0.15 mm

From a point source, objects are easily resolved as separate on the film. However, with increasing focal spot size, the radiation comes from all parts of the source. The radiation creating the image does not provide a sharp image but has blurring at the edges. If the objects are too close together they can appear as one or an extra 'object' can be created.

2) Compression

Typical compression force is 100 - 150 N

The compression force:
- Lowers patient radiation dose as the attenuation of the compressed breast is lower and a lower exposure can be used
- Reduces scatter as the breast is less thick so there is less probability of scatter happening within the tissue
- Spreads the tissues out so that there is less overlaying of features
- Reduces geometric unsharpness by moving some tissue closer to the image receptor
- Reduces movement unsharpness by holding the breast still
- The compressed breast is of more uniform attenuation

3) Anti-Scatter Grids

In mammography, moving grids are used for all contact (broad focus) images. For magnification images, using a fine focal spot size or an air gap technique is used to reduce the amount of scattered radiation reaching the receptor meaning a grid is not required.

Altering Parameters

Parameters need to be altered to provide optimal imaging of different breasts. Two factors need to be taken into consideration:

1. Thickness of breast
2. Composition of breast

1) Thickness

In large breasts:
- More radiation absorbed - higher doses needed
- More scatter
- Increased beam hardening (lower contrast)
- Longer exposure needed at 28 kV MoMo, therefore, movement artefacts may occur

Thinnest breasts: MoMo at 25 kV

Thickest breasts: MoRh or even WRh for very thick breasts at 32 kV

2) Composition

With more dense breasts, higher doses are needed due to extra attenuation and more beam hardening. Due to beam hardening, the AEC may cut off the exposure prematurely (the measured exposure will be of a higher intensity). To ensure this doesn't happen, one of two methods may be used:

1. A pre-exposure determines whether the breast is as dense as expected for this thickness by looking at the dose rate and beam hardening.
2. Adjustment on dose rate based on measuring the dose detected at the start of the examination and then adjusting the dose and exposure time as necessary.

Tomosynthesis

Superimposed tissue can mask pathology and, often, the pathology in breast disease can be very subtle. Breast tomography uses digital radiography to reconstruct planar images of sections of the breast. There are two main methods of acquiring breast tomosynthesis:

1. The x-ray tube traverses along an arc acquiring images as it travels and the detector remains stationary
2. The x-ray tube traverses along an arc and the detector also rotates

The images are then reconstructed using filtered back projection or iterative reconstruction (see 3.3 - Acquiring an Image (part 2)).

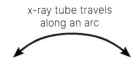

x-ray tube travels
along an arc

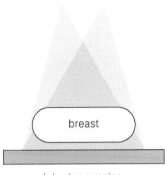

breast

detector remains
stationary

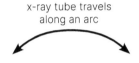

x-ray tube travels
along an arc

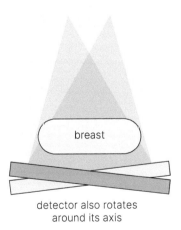

breast

detector also rotates
around its axis

Figure 46   Tomosynthesis

Pros
- Provides enhanced lesion detection
- Reduces false positive recalls
- Allows more precise lesion localisation

Cons
- Higher radiation dose (approximately double)
- High contrast objects (e.g. surgical clips) can cause significant artefacts
- Longer interpretation time
- Requires substantially more data storage

Summary

- Angled tube head
  - Cathode over chest wall (thickest part of breast) to exploit anode heel effect (higher energy radiation at thickest part of breast)
- Focus-to-film distance
  - Fixed at 65-66cm
- Target-filter material
  - General use - MoMo at 25 kV
  - Dense breasts - MoRh or RhRh at 32 kV
- Compression
  - Maximum pressure of 200N
  - Lowers patient radiation dose
  - Reduces scatter
  - Spreads the tissues out so that there is less overlaying of features
  - Reduces geometric unsharpness

- Reduces movement unsharpness
- More uniform attenuation
- Anti-scatter grids used
  - Except in magnification view where air-gap used
- Focal spot
  - Broad focal spot size = 0.3 mm
  - Fine focus focal spot size = 0.1 to 0.15 mm
- Breast tomosynthesis
  - X-ray tube travels in an arc +/- detector rotates
  - Allows reconstruction of planar images
  - Pros:
    - Reduced recall rate
    - Increased detection of pathology
    - More precise lesion localisation
  - Cons:
    - Increased radiation dose (double)
    - High contrast objects cause significant artefacts
    - Longer interpretation times
    - More data storage required

2.7 Fluoroscopy

Fluoroscopy is the use of real time x-ray imaging. It used to utilise image intensifiers, which have been in use since the late 1950's, but now uses flat panel detectors, which are similar to the digital radiography used in projection radiology.

1) Definitions

Fluoroscopy
- Real time imaging viewed on a display monitor in the clinical room
- Matrix is smaller (512 × 512 pixels) and 8 bits of grey scale only needed as temporal, not spatial, resolution is prioritised
- Can acquire continuous (cine) or pulsed fluorographic images

Fluorography
- Images usually formed and viewed after the x-ray exposure is complete
- Better quality images acquired than in fluoroscopy but at higher doses
- Matrix is typically 1024 × 1024 pixels with each pixel representing 10 bits of grey scale information

'Greyscale' digital x-ray imaging modes
- e.g. fluoroscopy, digital cardiac and digital spot imaging in which the image is similar to a plain film radiograph or inverted.

Subtractive digital imaging
- e.g. angiography. Base image taken which is then subtracted from the image with contrast to result in an image showing the contrast only.

Image intensifier (II)

The IITV system is characterised by the ability to convert the input light into a much higher output (gain or intensification). The x-ray II tube is a vacuum glass or ceramic envelope surrounded by a metal housing (to shield from external light sources and magnetic fields).

The degree to which an image is intensified (or amplified) is given by the **brightness gain** ($G_{brightness}$) which is the ratio of the brightness of the output screen compared to the input screen.

$$G_{brightness} = G_{minification} \times G_{flux}$$

Where: $G_{minification}$ = minification gain
G_{flux} = flux gain

In turn, the minification gain describes how much the brightness has increased due to the demagnification of the image in the II tube.

$$G_{minification} = (D_{input} / D_{output})^2$$

Where: D_{input} = diameter of the input screen
D_{output} = diameter of the output screen

In measuring the ability of the II tube to amplify the signal we are unable to measure the brightness of the input screen, which limits the use of the $G_{brightness}$. Instead we now use the image intensifier conversion factor (G_x).

$$G_x = L / X'$$

Where: L = luminance of the II output (units = candelas m^{-2})
X' = II entrance dose rate (units = μGy s^{-1})

Factors that affect the brightness gain of an II tube:
- Magnification -
  - The demagnification (i.e. minimising) electron-optical factor. More demagnification = higher gain
  - Zoom field: G_x falls in proportion to the reduction in the area of the input field
- Flux -
  - Higher voltage difference applied across II tube = more flux gain

Some numbers:
- $G_{minification}$ ~ 100
- G_{flux} ~ 100
- G_x ~ 10-30

2) Configuration of equipment

- Standard radiography/fluoroscopy (R/F):
  - Under table x-ray tube with an over-couch II system
  - Table can be tilted and rotated
  - Radiologist stands beside patient to operate system
- Remote control R/F:
  - X-ray tube mounted over the bed and II system underneath
  - Higher scattered dose so radiologist has to stand behind screen to operate system via remote control
- Fixed C-arm:
  - II x-ray tube and II system attached to a C-structure that allows it to be rotated around and moved up and down patient as required
  - Can be ceiling or floor mounted
- Mobile C-arm:
  - System that can be transported on wheels to where it is needed e.g. theatres

3) Image intensifier system (IITV)

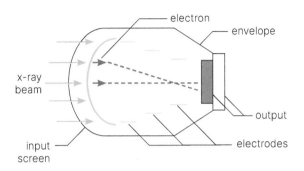

Figure 47   II system

Internal construction of an II x-ray tube:

1. Input screen
2. Electron-optics
3. Output stage

1) Input screen

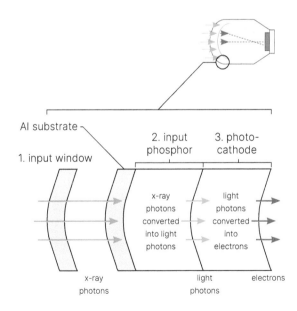

Figure 48   Input screen of II tube

II input window

▪ Convex metal shield that covers the input face of the II

▪ Usually made of aluminium or titanium foil (low Z metal) to allow x-ray beam to enter with minimum attenuation

▪ Provides protection for sensitive input components of the tube and maintains the vacuum

Input phosphor

▪ Layer of **sodium activated caesium iodide (CsI:Na)** for good x-ray absorption efficiency (70-90%)

▪ Channelled into tiny needle-like crystals (5μm in diameter) with fibreoptic-like characteristics

▪ Deposited on a thin aluminium substrate

▪ CsI:Na usually 400-500μm thick

▪ Each x-ray photon produces ~3000 light photons in the **blue spectrum**

Photocathode

▪ Fluorescent emission from phosphor then absorbed in a light-activated photocathode comprising a very thin layer of **antimony caesium (SbCs3)** alloy that has a spectral sensitivity well matched to the blue light emission of CsI:Na

▪ Absorption of the fluorescent light photons releases a pattern of electrons in the body of the II tube

▪ Approximately 200 electrons released per absorbed x-ray photon

2) II electron optics

The input screen is maintained at a negative voltage with respect to the anode (output screen) with a potential difference of 25 kV. This means the electrons produced are accelerated across the II tube and carefully focused on the output screen. The output screen is 1/10 the diameter of the input screen and, therefore, a minified and inverted image is produced.

Electron Focusing

Focusing electrodes are metal rings within the tube that are held at positive voltages with respect to the photocathode. This constrains the electrons in the tube to travel along paths that lead them directly to the output screen, such that the pattern of electron intensities falling on the screen are an exact (but minified) replica of the pattern intensities on the input screen.

Magnification

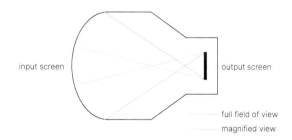

Figure 49   Magnification in fluoroscopy

Magnification is achieved electronically with electronic focusing of the electron beam. If a smaller area of the input screen is sampled the image is still shown on the same area of output screen (the output image size remains constant). This results in a magnified image. Because less signal is used, the image is less bright and, therefore, a higher dose is needed. However, as the image magnified, the resolution is better.

Magnification causes:
- Less bright image and increased dose required
- Better resolution

3) II Output Stage

Output Screen

Thin layer of **silver-activated zinc cadmium sulphide (ZnCdS:Ag)** crystals deposited on the inner surface of the output window that convert the electrons into light photons. The output image is intensified significantly by the acceleration of the electrons and the minification of the image that occurs in the II tube. The screen is normally 25-35 mm in diameter and a few micrometres thick.

This inner surface of the output screen is coated in a very thin layer of **aluminium** that:
- Forms part of the anode structure
- High speed electrons travel through the aluminium layer
- The layer is opaque preventing the light emitted by the phosphor from back-illuminating the photocathode and degrading II performance. The light is reflected back towards the output increasing the gain of the II tube.

Output Window

This is an optically transparent glass block port through which the intensified light image exits the II tube. Scatter of light, or halation, in the output window can seriously degrade the contrast of the II output image. Minimising halation can be done with:

- Smoked glass
- Special optical coatings
- Very thick glass
- Fibre-optic bundle

4) Summary

1. X-ray photons enter tube through aluminium or titanium window
2. Hit input phosphor layer of sodium activated caesium iodide and release light photons
3. Light photons detected by photocathode that then release electrons into the tube
4. Electrons accelerated and focused onto the output screen (silver-activated zinc cadmium sulphide crystals) as a minified and inverted image
5. Light photons released that then leave through the output window

Display of Image

The image from the output screen is displayed on a monitor using a TV imaging system.

1) II TV camera

These are no longer used in clinical practice.

Electronic TV camera tube

A TV camera tube uses an electron beam that scans across, line by line. The scanning direction is determined by focusing and deflection coils arranged around the outside of the tube.

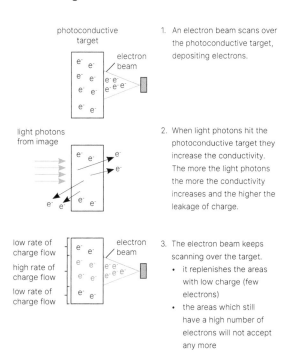

1. An electron beam scans over the photoconductive target, depositing electrons.

2. When light photons hit the photoconductive target they increase the conductivity. The more the light photons the more the conductivity increases and the higher the leakage of charge.

3. The electron beam keeps scanning over the target.
   - it replenishes the areas with low charge (few electrons)
   - the areas which still have a high number of electrons will not accept any more

4. The flow of charge through a resistor creates a voltage. This is the video signal (time-varying video voltage signal).

Figure 50 II TV camera

Determining resolution:

- Vertical resolution is determined by the number of scan lines
- Horizontal resolution is determined by the

bandwidth of the system (higher bandwidth = lower resolution)

2) Charged coupled device (CCD) sensors

Solid state CCD sensors are superseding the electronic TV camera tube. Each pixel in the CCD has an associated electrode. A positive bias voltage is applied to the electrode that forms a "potential well" in the region of the silicon substrate.

1. The light photons (from the II output) are absorbed into the silicon substrate of the CCD (light-sensitive array)
2. Each light photon gives rise to an electron-hole pair
   - The positive "hole" drains away
   - The negative electrons accumulate in a potential well
3. These charge packages are then transferred to the light shielded storage array
4. The data is then read from the storage section line-by-line
   - The quantity of electronic charge which accumulates at each pixel is directly proportional to the intensity of the incident light

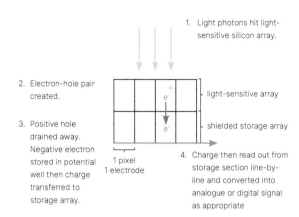

1. Light photons hit light-sensitive silicon array.

2. Electron-hole pair created.

3. Positive hole drained away. Negative electron stored in potential well then charge transferred to storage array.

1 pixel
1 electrode

light-sensitive array

shielded storage array

4. Charge then read out from storage section line-by-line and converted into analogue or digital signal as appropriate

Figure 51   Charged coupled device

Benefits

- Small, inexpensive, compact, low-power consumption
- Self-scanning image readout
- Negligible lag (important for video fluoroscopy)
- Excellent thermal, electrical and magnetic stability
- Excellent serviceability and long life-time
- Compatibility with digital x-ray imaging modalities

Image Quality

1) Automatic brightness control (ABC)

Aka automatic dose rate control. The purpose of the ABC is to maintain constant viewing condition independent of examination. This is done by mA and kV regulation. The need to alter the mA or kV is determined by either electronically sampling the video signal or by measuring the II light output with a photo-sensor.

The allowable dose allowed by the ABC is determined by the mode used:

- Minimum patient dose rate mode
- Standard patient dose rate mode
- High patient dose rate mode (high image quality)

N.B. ABC is used in fluoroscopy, automatic exposure control (AEC) is used in fluorography and radiography.

2) Digital image processing

To improve the appearance of the image on the screen there are several algorithms that can be applied to the digital image.

Greyscale processing

- Greyscale range compression
- Used to suppress or highlight intensities and improve contrast balance of image. Achieved by using either an analogue (video) circuit or via a look-up-table (LUT)
- Contrast and brightness adjustment

Spatial filtering

- Similar to edge enhancement in projection radiography
- Improves displayed spatial resolution
- Best used for high contrast image e.g. barium GI studies

Temporal filtering

- This is used to decrease the level of noise
- The current frame is averaged with a set of the preceding frames. This creates a digitally generated lag to smooth the noise fluctuations. Also, the higher signal created by combining several frames results in a smaller proportion of noise
- This is best used for structures that are quasi-static

Flat Panel Detector

Flat panel detectors utilise the same technology as digital radiography in that there is a flat panel of detectors that provide a direct electronic readout instead of requiring the conversion of analogue to digital as is seen in the IITV. Similar to digital radiography dynamic FP detectors can be direct or indirect. However, they are more commonly indirect with a CsI:Tl x-ray scintillator layer which is superimposed onto an a-Si high resolution active matrix.

Benefits

- Smaller equipment
- Video signal emerges in digital form, reducing electronic noise
- Square or rectangular field (unlike circular field in IITV) = better coverage in the corners
- Better temporal resolution with matrix size of 2048 × 2048 pixels
- Greyscale of 12 or 14 bits per pixel

- Produces better quality images than IITV
- Fewer artefacts such as geometrical distortion, vignetting or contrast loss
- Detective quantum efficiency 10-20% better than IITV so can afford to reduce patient dose
- Zoom option available (but doesn't increase spatial resolution as it does in IITV)

Digital Subtraction Angiography

A common procedure performed using fluoroscopy is a digital subtraction angiography (DSA). In this procedure the contrast outlined structure is highlighted by removing the background anatomical structures from the images. This is done in four stages:

1. Acquire mask image (I_M) to record anatomical background
2. Contrast injected. Series of images acquired which show arrival and run-off of contrast (contrast medium enhanced image, I_c)
3. Image frames subtracted via digital processor. Any structures that are common to set 1 and set 2 are subtracted (i.e. all background anatomy but not the contrast filled structures)
4. Amplify contrast signal to boost displayed contrast of the vessels

1) Artefacts

The artefact most unique to DSA is **misregistration**

- The movement of a structure by even 1 mm can cause misregistration.
- These are corrected by the computer with:
  - Pixel shifting (contrast and mask images spatially offset prior to subtraction to compensate for movement) and
  - Remasking (re-mask to an image later in the run-off phase instead of the initial mask)

Dose

1) Dose to patient

The dose to the patient is better represented by the skin dose rate i.e. the dose per unit of time.

Maximum entrance skin dose rate limit 100 mGy per minute

IITV patient entrance skin dose	3 to 10 mGy per minute 10 to 30 mGy per minute for larger patient
Digital fluoroscopy	10 - 40 nGy per frame at II entrance
Digital cardiac image acquisition	Dose per frame 10x higher than fluoroscopy

Digital spot imaging (fluorography)	Dose 100x higher than fluoroscopy
Subtractive digital fluorography (e.g. angiography)	Dose 1000x higher than fluoroscopy

Minimising patient dose
- Setup of equipment
  - Tight collimation of x-ray beam
  - Appropriate x-ray beam spectral filter to minimise patient skin dose rate
  - Increase distance between patient and x-ray source
  - Minimise gap between patient and II entrance
  - Remove anti-scatter grid if possible
- Imaging procedure
  - Avoid constantly imaging at same projection angle
  - Minimise x-ray beam on time
  - ABC mode with lowest dose rate possible for diagnostic images
  - Pulsed fluoroscopy with minimum acceptable pulse rate if possible
  - Avoid use of II zoom
- Digital processes
  - Last-image-hold
  - Road mapping - digital fluorographic image acquired during contrast injection phase. This image is then subtracted from subsequent fluoroscopy images in real time to highlight the contrast-injected structure and remove the background anatomy
- **Fluoroscopy**
  - Maximise concentration of contrast medium in vessel of interest, e.g. in-

tra-arterial rather than intra-venous, to increase signal and therefore enable lower dose

2) Dose to staff

- Stray radiation:
  - Leakage of from tube housing should be less than 1 mGy per hour at 1 metre from the focus
  - Scatter of x-rays from patient is the most significant contribution to staff dose. ~0.1% of patient dose at 1m distance
  - Secondary scatter of x-rays from structures in the room

Minimising staff dose
- Use of lead aprons and other radiation shields e.g. gloves, glasses and thyroid protection
- Lead-rubber drapes and movable lead glass shields
- Maintain maximum possible distance from patient
- Monitor individual staff doses

Summary

1) Definitions:

- Fluoroscopy: Real-time imaging viewed on display monitor in clinical room. Higher temporal but lower spatial resolution than fluorography

- Fluorography: Image displayed after x-ray exposure
- Fluorography and fluoroscopy imaged using image intensifier system (IITV) or, more recently, digital flat panel detectors (FP detector)

2) IITV system

Measuring intensification

- Calculations
  - Brightness gain = minification gain x flux gain
  - Minification gain = $(D_{input} / D_{output})^2$ (where D is diameter of input and output screen respectively)
  - Image intensifier conversion factor $(G_x) = L / X'$ (where L = luminance of II output, X' = II entrance dose rate)
- Factors that affect brightness gain
  - More minimisation = higher gain
  - G_x falls in proportion to the reduction in the area of the input field in zoom setting
  - Higher voltage applied across II tube = more flux gain

II x-ray tube

- Input screen
  - II input window: aluminium or titanium foil to allow x-rays to enter tube and maintain vacuum
- Input phosphor

Layer of CsI:Na for good x-ray absorption efficiency. Each x-ray photon produces ~3000 light photons in blue spectrum

- Photocathode
  - Fluorescent emission from phosphor absorbed by light-activated photo-cathode made of SbCs3 which then releases electrons into body of II tube

II electron optics

- Input screen at negative charge compared to output screen to direct electron towards output screen.
- Electron focusing: positively charged electrodes along tube direct electron path to create exact but minified and inverted image on input screen
- Magnification: achieved via electronically focusing electron beam. Magnified images use less signal and so need a higher dose but improve the resolution

II output

- Output screen made of thin layer of ZnCdS:Ag that convert electrons into light photos that then leave through the output window

3) Display of image

II TV camera

- Electronic TV camera uses electron beam that scans across photoconductive target to create flow of electrons, the rate of which corresponds to the amount of light photons striking that area

Charged coupled device (CCD sensors)
- Now more commonly used
- Each pixel has an associated electrode. The accumulation of charge is directly proportional to the intensity of the incident light
- Flat panel detector
  - Utilises same technology as digital radiography
  - Most commonly indirect dynamic FP detector with CsI:Tl x-ray scintillator layer superimposed onto a-Si high resolution active matrix

4) Image quality

- Automatic brightness control (ABC, fluoroscopy) (c.f. automatic exposure control, AEC, fluorography)
  - Alters kV and mA to ensure stable quality of images. This, in turn, alters the patient dose
  - Done by measuring II light output with a photo-sensor or electronically sampling video signal
- Digital processing
  - Grey scale processing with greyscale range compression: suppress or highlight intensities and improve contrast balance. Uses analogue (video) circuit or via a look-up-table (LUT)
  - Spatial filtering: similar to edge enhancement in projection radiography. Improves displayed spatial resolution
  - Temporal filtering: decreases level of dose by summing current image with previous frames, averaging out signal and resulting in smaller proportion of noise

5) Dose

- Patient dose
  - Measured in skin dose rates
- Staff dose
  - Greatest contribution to staff dose is from scatter, amounts to ~0.1% of patient dose at a distance of 1m

3

This chapter focuses on the techniques of CT imaging and will cover the equipment used to acquire an image, how the image is formed and displayed, the factors affecting the quality of the image and how dose is measured.

3.1	CT Equipment	79
3.2	Acquiring an Image (Part 1)	85
3.3	Acquiring an Image (Part 2)	90
3.4	Dual-Energy CT	93
3.5	CT Image Quality	97
3.6	CT Artefacts	103
3.7	CT Dose	110

3.1 CT Equipment

Components

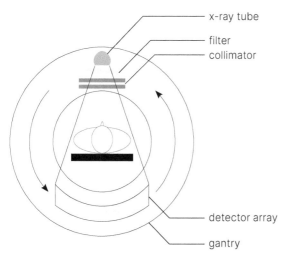

Figure 52 CT machine

1) Filter

Placed between the x-ray source and the patient (similar to that used in plain film radiography).

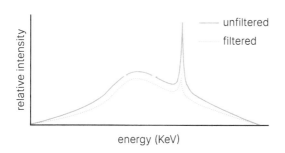

Figure 53 The x-ray beam intensity through a filter

1. Removes low energy (soft) x-rays that do not contribute to image formation but do increase patient dose.

2. As the low energy x-rays are removed there is a narrower spectrum of x-ray energies creating a more "monochromatic" beam. Image reconstruction is based upon the assumption of a single energy, monochromatic beam.

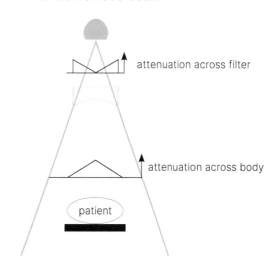

Figure 54 Bow-tie filter

3. In some scanners the filter is shaped to shape the beam e.g. "bow-tie" filter. The lateral edges of a body are thinner than the centre causing less attenuation of the x-ray beam. A shaped filter compensates for this by attenuating the lateral edges of the beam more than the centre. These filters come in different shapes/sizes depending on the body part imaged. A bow-tie filter, as shown in the diagram above, is designed for imaging the chest or abdomen. If the head was being imaged then a smaller filter would be used, to match the size of the head.

2) Collimator

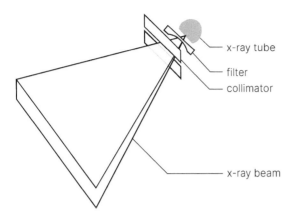

Figure 55   Collimator of a CT machine

The Collimator is placed between the filter and the patient.
1. Lowers radiation dose to patient
2. Restricts scatter from outside of desired slice

3) Detector Array

The original single-slice scanners had one row of detectors. Now all scanners are multi-slice and have 8-64 rows of detectors. There are generally 1000-2000 detectors in each row.

Important properties for detectors
- High detection efficiency for x-rays in CT energy range
- High dynamic range
- Narrow gaps between active elements (good geometrical efficiency)
- Fast response
- Low cost
- Small physical size

Types of detectors
1. Solid state detector (SSD)

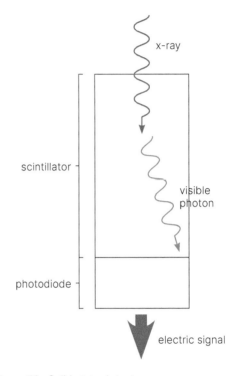

Figure 56   Solid state detector

There is a solid scintillator layer that converts the x-rays into visible light photons. The photodiode then converts the photon input into an electrical signal. This is the most commonly used detector.

Properties:
- High detection efficiency (~90%)
- High geometrical efficiency (~80%)
- Small physical size of detector elements

2. Ionisation chamber detector (no longer used)

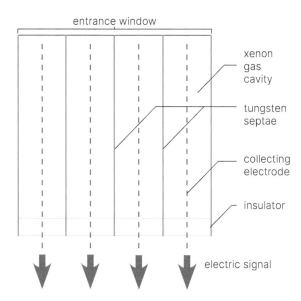

entrance window

xenon gas cavity

tungsten septae

collecting electrode

insulator

electric signal

Figure 57   Ionisation chamber detector

The detector array is a single vessel filled with gases of a high atomic number (Krypton / Xenon) and subdivided into separate detectors by tungsten septae.

The x-rays ionise the gas and produce a signal at the collection electrodes.

Properties:
- Lower detection efficiency (~50%)
- High stability
- Consistent sensitivity between detector elements

Ionisation chambers have been superseded by solid-state detectors and are no longer used as they are unsuitable for multislice scanners.

4) Gantry

A slip-ring enables continuous rotation of the CT scanner gantry. Brushes on the rotating gantry, through contact with the stationary ring, allows power to be supplied to the gantry and the signal to be passed to the computer. Rotation times are between 0.25 - 3 seconds.

Generations of CT Scanner

1) First generation

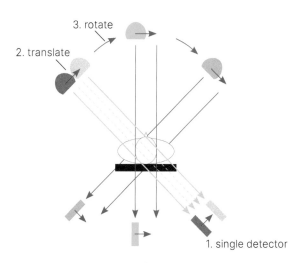

3. rotate

2. translate

1. single detector

Figure 58   1st generation of CT machine

Translate-Rotate
1. The x-ray beam is picked-up by a single detector.
2. The x-ray source and detector then move together (**translate**)
3. The two then **rotate** together to image a different angle

4. This is repeated until a single slice is scanned
5. The two then move down the patient to start imaging a different slice

This method took 5 minutes per slice to scan

2) Second generation

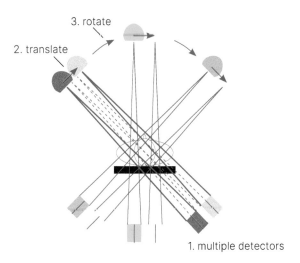

Figure 59   2ⁿᵈ generation of CT machine

Translate-Rotate

1. The x-ray beam is picked-up by a row of up to 30 detectors.
2. The x-ray source and detector then move together (**translate**)
3. The two then **rotate** together to image a different angle
4. This is repeated until a single slice is scanned
5. The two then move down the patient to start imaging a different slice in the patient

This method took 5-90 seconds per slice

3) Third generation

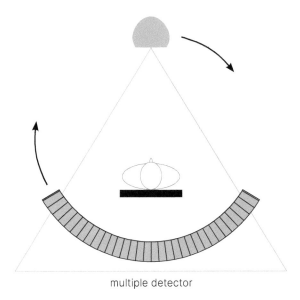

Figure 60   3ʳᵈ generation of CT machine

Rotate-Rotate

1. The x-ray beam hits a row of detectors wide enough to image the whole slice
2. The two then **rotate** together to image a different angle
3. This is repeated until a single slice is scanned then the array is moved to a different slice (axial scanning). Alternatively, the detector array is continually moved down the patient as it rotates (spiral scanning), see 3.2 - Acquiring an Image (Part 1).

This is the **most commonly used method today** and takes about 0.3 seconds to image a single slice

4) Fourth generation

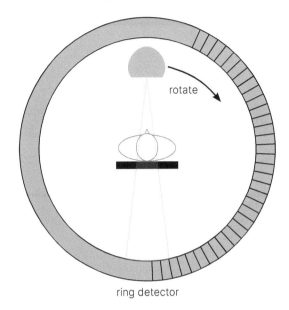

ring detector

Figure 61   4th generation of CT machine

Rotate-fixed

1. There is a fixed complete ring of detectors
2. The x-ray source rotates around to capture a slice
3. Both then move down the patient to begin imaging a different slice

This is not commonly used today.

5) Electron Beam Scanner

(Sometimes described as 5th generation CT).

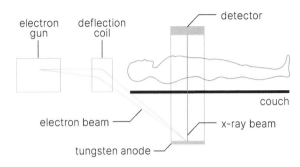

Figure 62   5th generation of CT machine

▪ An electron beam is deflected by an electromagnetic field onto a fixed array of tungsten anode target underneath the patient.
▪ The electromagnetic field sweeps the electron beam across the target creating hundreds of x-ray beams firing through the patient to the detector above the patient.
▪ Fast scanning of 50-250 milliseconds.
▪ Mainly used for certain cardiac imaging.

Summary

1) Components of a CT scanner:

Filter:
▪ Placed between x-ray source and patient
▪ Removes low energy x-rays
▪ Produces a more monochromatic beam
▪ May be bowtie-shaped to even out atten-

uation once it passes through the body

Collimator:
- Placed between filter and patient
- Narrows beam to produce thinner slice
- Less scatter from outside of the slice
- Lower patient dose

Detector array:
- Solid state:
    - Most commonly used
    - Solid scintillator layer converts x-rays into light photons
- Ionisation chamber detector (no longer used):
    - Gas filled single chamber that is ionised by x-rays passing through

Gantry:
- Slip-ring system allows continuous rotation of the gantry

2) Generations of CT scanners:

- 1st: Translate-Rotate with single detector
- 2nd: Translate-Rotate with row of detectors
- 3rd: Rotate-Rotate with continuous rotation of a row of detectors. Most commonly used CT type
- 4th: Rotate-Fixed with complete ring of fixed detectors
- 5th: Electron beam scanner used in cardiac imaging

3.2   Acquiring an Image (Part 1)

This section covers the role of the physical equipment in acquiring an image i.e. the gantry and detectors.

Axial vs Spiral Scanning

2) Spiral scanning

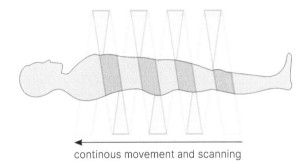

continous movement and scanning

Figure 64   Spiral scanning

1) Axial scanning

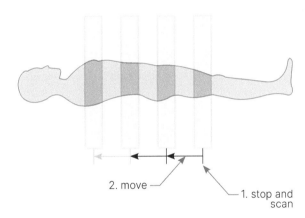

2. move

1. stop and scan

Figure 63   Axial scanning

"Step and shoot"
1. Gantry stops and rotates to acquire data from single slice
2. X-rays switched off
3. Patient moves to next slice
4. Rotates to acquire data from next slice

- **Also known as** helical scanning
- Gantry keeps rotating continuously releasing x-ray beams.
- The couch simultaneously moves.
- This results in a continuous spiral scanning pattern.

Advantages:
- Avoids respiratory misregistration as scan performed during one breath
- More effective use of contrast agent as faster scanning enables scanning during multiple phases in one contrast injection e.g. portal venous, angiographic, delayed
- Overlapping slices allows better reconstruction and helps in showing smaller lesions
- Pitch > 1 can be used to reduce scan time and / or radiation dose and still cover the same volume

All images are now acquired in this way.

…measure of overlap during scan.

$$\text{Pitch} = \text{distance couch travels} / \text{width of slice}$$

$$\text{Pitch} = 20/10 = 2$$

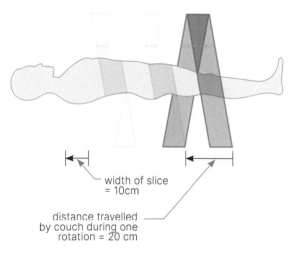

width of slice
= 10cm

distance travelled
by couch during one
rotation = 20 cm

Figure 65   CT scanner pitch of 2

$$\text{Pitch} = 10/10 = 1$$

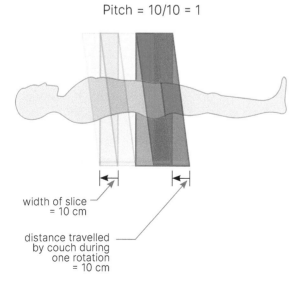

width of slice
= 10 cm

distance travelled
by couch during
one rotation
= 10 cm

Figure 66   CT scanner pitch of 1

$$\text{Pitch} = 5/10 = 0.5$$

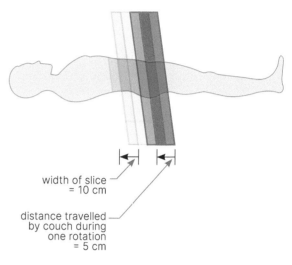

width of slice
= 10 cm

distance travelled
by couch during
one rotation
= 5 cm

Figure 67   CT scanner pitch of 0.5

- A pitch number **1** = couch travels **more than the width of the beam** i.e. there are gaps
- A pitch number **< 1** = couch travels **less than the width of the beam** i.e. there is overlap

For higher pitch numbers:
- Advantages:
  - Lower radiation dose
  - Quicker scan
- Disadvantages:
  - More sparsely sampled

Multislice Scanning

Rather than just have one row of detectors, we now have multiple parallel rows of detectors. Certain rows of detectors can then be selected to change the slice thickness along with the collimator.

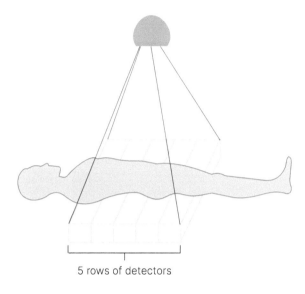

5 rows of detectors

Figure 68   Multiple detector rows

Advantages:
- Faster scanning due to wider total active detector width
- Better dynamic imaging due to faster scanning times
- Thinner slices
- 3D imaging is enabled by thin slices
- Simultaneous acquisition of multiple slices

3) Detector arrays

Types of Multislice Detector Types:
1. Linear
2. Adaptive
3. Hybrid arrays

1. Linear array

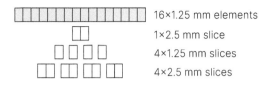

Figure 69   Linear detector array

- All the rows of the detectors are the same width.

2. Adaptive array

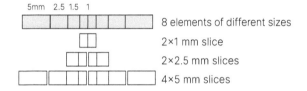

Figure 70   Adaptive detector array

- The elements within the central detector rows are the thinnest and they get wider towards the outside.
- **Advantages:**
  - As few detector elements as possible activated to still give a large range of detector slices.
  - Fewer detector rows activated means fewer septae dividing up the rows. This improves the dose efficiency.
- **Disadvantage:**
  - Upgrading to more data channels requires an expensive detector replacement.

3. Hybrid array

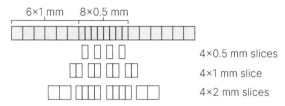

Figure 71 Hybrid detector array

- Similar to linear arrays in that the elements within the detector rows are the same width across. However, the central group of detector rows are narrower than the outer rows.
- These are the main detector arrays used for 16-slice scanners and above.

4) Multislice pitch

There are two methods to calculate the pitch in a multislice scanner. The first (pitch$_d$) is analogous to the single slice pitch and only takes into account the width of the x-ray beam.

$$Pitch_d = couch\ travel\ per\ rotation\ /\ width\ of\ x\text{-}ray\ beam$$

However, this does not fully represent the overlapping of the x-ray beam and, instead, pitch$_x$ is now used.

$$Pitch_x = couch\ travel\ per\ rotation\ /\ total\ width\ of\ simultaneously\ acquired\ slices$$

This is comparable to the definition of pitch for single slice spiral scanning as the total collimated width is analogous to the detector subgroup width in single slice spiral scanning.

Key Points

- Pitch
    - Single slice pitch = detector pitch = couch travel per rotation / detector width
    - Multislice pitch = beam pitch = couch travel per rotation / total width of simultaneously acquired slices
- Slice thickness
    - Single slice CT = determined by collimation. Limited by detector row width
    - Multisclice CT = determined by width of detector rows

Summary

- Spiral scanning now used instead of axial scanning
- Pitch = distance couch travels / width of beam
    - Pitch > 1 means there are gaps between slices
    - Pitch = 1 means there is no beam overlap
    - Pitch < 1 means the beam overlaps

1) Multislice scanning

Multislice scanning uses lots of rows and each row consists of equal sized detectors

- Rows combined to give different number of slices. Number of slices limited by number of data channels.
- Older scanners may use one of the following types of detector array:
  - Linear array: all detector rows are of equal width
  - Adaptive array: detector rows are of different widths
  - Hybrid array: central rows narrower than outer rows. Most commonly used array today.

Multislice pitch

- $Pitch_x$ = distance couch travels / total width of slices
- $Pitch_d$ = distance couch travels / detector subgroup width

3.3 Acquiring an Image (Part 2)

This section covers the processing aspect of acquiring an image.

Physics

A CT image is made up of pixels along a grey-scale. What determines the level of grey is the density of the material, also expressed as the linear attenuation coefficient, and this is represented numerically by the Hounsfield Units (also called the CT number). The Hounsfield units are set so that water measures 0 and everything else is relative to this.

$$HU = 1000 \times (\mu t - \mu w) / \mu w$$

Where:
μt = attenuation coefficient of tissue
μw = attenuation coefficient of water

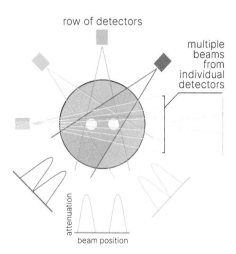

Figure 72   Summed linear attenuation coefficient

Each detector in the CT scanner samples a line of the patient and the sum total of the attenuation of the material passed through along the beam path is calculated. As the gantry rotates the detectors receive beams at different angles so, in the end, we have a series of values of summed linear attenuation coefficients from different angles. Now, these need to be processed to form an image.

1) Typical Hounsfield unit values

Tissue	CT number (HU)
Bone	+1000
Liver	40 to 60
White matter	20 to 30
Grey matter	37 to 45
Intravascular blood	30 to 45
Fresh clotted blood	70 to 80
Muscle	10 to 40
Kidney	30
CSF	15
Water	0
Fat	-50 to -100
Air	-1000

Post-Processing

1) Backprojection

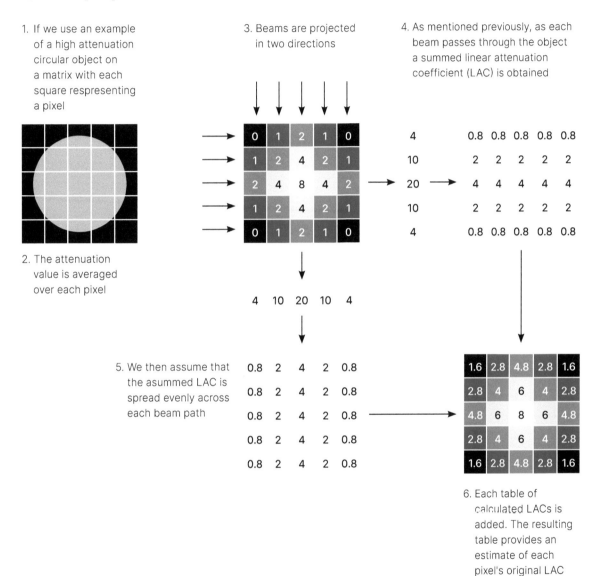

1. If we use an example of a high attenuation circular object on a matrix with each square respresenting a pixel

2. The attenuation value is averaged over each pixel

3. Beams are projected in two directions

4. As mentioned previously, as each beam passes through the object a summed linear attenuation coefficient (LAC) is obtained

5. We then assume that the asummed LAC is spread evenly across each beam path

6. Each table of calculated LACs is added. The resulting table provides an estimate of each pixel's original LAC

Figure 73   Backprojection technique

There are a few main issues with backprojection:

1. Too few projections cause artefacts in the image as there are too few directions of summed LACs to accurately represent the image. Typically 2000 projections are used.

2. Even with a large number of projections

the edges of structures are not well delineated due to the averaging out of values and there is blurring caused by the backprojection technique. This is corrected with **filtered backprojection**.

2) Iterative Reconstruction

This is generally a more time-consuming method but is proving useful for low dose CT studies.

It involves several steps:

1. Filtered backprojection is initially performed.
2. The computer then calculates what it expected the detectors to have received based on the image generated THEN works out the difference between the actual detector measurements and the calculated measurements. It then uses this information to generate an updated image.
3. This continues through multiple iterations, each time bringing the calculated values closer and closer to the true values.

Summary

- Image is made up of pixels of varying grey, the shade of which is assigned a "Hounsfield Unit" (also called "CT number") which is compared to a look-up-table to give the greyscale.
- The x-ray beam and detectors rotate around the subject sampling rows at different angles. Each row is coded as a single summed attenuation value.
- The attenuation values are then processed to produce the image mainly via two techniques
  - **Backprojection:** The summed attenuation values are averaged out over the row. With several projections it comes closer to actual image. There are some weaknesses:
    - Too few projections cause artefacts
    - Blurred images - solved by filtered backprojection
    - For multislice scanners filter interpolation is used in which all projections within a certain axial slice are summed and averaged.
  - **Iterative reconstruction:** Filtered backprojection is initially performed to assign a number value to all pixels in the matrix. The computer then calculates what it expected the detectors to have received based on the image generated and compares this to the actual detector measurements, adjusting the image values to bring them closer to the true values.
    - Almost exclusively used now.
    - **Weakness:** Calculations are lengthy
    - **Strength:** Reducing CT dose

3.4 Dual-Energy CT

The image from a CT study is a representation of the total attenuation per voxel within the imaged subject. Dual-energy CT (DECT) utilises the photoelectric effect to separate out different materials within the voxel based upon their different attenuations at different beam energies.

The photoelectric effect, as we've mentioned before, is the ejection by a photon of an electron from the innermost K-shell of an atom. An electron from the next shell fills the empty space. The energy from this is released in the form of a photoelectron. The photoelectric event can only occur if the incident photon has enough energy to overcome the binding energy of the electrons within the K-shell.

When the incident photon has an energy just above the K-shell binding energy there is a sudden jump in attenuation (K-edge) because of the increased photoelectric absorption. The K-shell binding energy and, therefore, the K-edge, depends on the element and it increases as the atomic number increases.

We can analyse the attenuation of material over different beam energies to determine the constituents of that material. As an example, if we have an element with a K-edge at 70 keV and one at 130 keV:

Substance	K Edge (keV)	Atomic Number (Z)
Hydrogen	0.01	1
Carbon	0.28	6
Nitrogen	0.40	7
Oxygen	0.53	8
Calcium	4.00	20
Iodine	33.20	53
Barium	37.45	56
Gadolinium	50.20	64

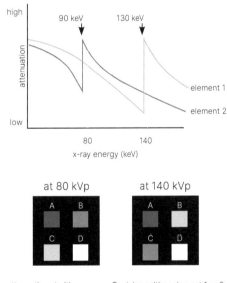

A - No attenuation at either energy. Contains neither element 1 or 2
B - Higher attenuation at 140 kVp. Higher concentration of element 1
C - Higher attenuation at 80 kVp. Higher concentration of element 2
D - Similar attenuation at both energies. Equal amounts of both

Figure 74   Dual energy imaging

Techniques

There are several ways to perform dual-energy CT.

Dual-source DECT

- Two x-ray tubes of different voltages with two sets of detectors paired to the x-ray tubes. The x-ray tubes are at 90° to each other.
- Pros:
    - Simultaneous acquisition and processing at the two energies leads to quicker acquisition, good overlap of images acquired at the two voltages.
    - Can independently optimise the signal-to-noise ratio for each x-ray tube-detector pair
- Cons:
    - Increased dosage (two scans acquired)
    - Scattered radiation from one tube may be detected by the detector for the other tube

Single-source DECT

- Single x-ray tube
- Many techniques as follows:

Single-source consecutive DECT

- Two helical scans acquired consecutively at different tube potentials followed by coregistration of images

- Motion can lead to poor overlap of each image
- Increased dosage (two scans acquired)

Single-source sequential DECT

- Each axial rotation (i.e. each slice) is performed at high- and then low-tube potential
- Increased dosage (two scans acquired) but less motion artefact
- Poorer temporal resolution as the patient is scanned twice

Single-source fast kilovoltage (kVp) switching DECT

- X-ray tube switches rapidly between high- and low-tube potential multiple times within the same rotation
- Lower dosage (one scan acquired)
- Requires very fast data sampling and may result in large overlap between high and low energies

Single-source twin-beam DECT

- Single x-ray tube and two material filter splits the x-ray beam into high-energy and low-energy spectra before it reaches the patient
- Simultaneous acquisition and processing at the two energies leads to quicker acquisition and excellent temporal resolution

Detector-based spectral CT

- Single x-ray tube with a single high tube potential beam
- Single detector but made of two layers (sandwich detector) that simultaneously detects two energies.
- Dual-energy analysis can be performed on every data set acquired.

Applications of DECT

Separate out materials

- Perfused blood volume / blood pool imaging e.g. pulmonary embolus and myocardial ischaemia
- Create virtual unenhanced images by removing iodine
- Atherosclerotic plaque removal
- Virtual non-calcium images - remove calcium to identify iodine uptake in bones i.e. bone marrow oedema
- Detect silicon from breast implant leakage

Hepatic

- Detection and characterisation of hepatic lesions - much more sensitive to enhancement within small hepatic lesions

Renal

- Distinguish hyperattenuating renal cysts from enhancing renal cell carcinoma
- Identify renal calculi within contrast-filled renal collecting system
- Characterise composition of renal calculi - specifically differentiating between uric acid containing and non-uric acid containing stones

Oncology

- Increased lesion conspicuity = better delineation of margins = more accurate size measurements
- Iodine maps can differentiate bland thrombus from tumour
- Better assessment of response to treatment

Vascular imaging

- Lower kVp is closer to K-edge of iodine than the 120 kVp used in normal imaging i.e. can use lower dose of contrast and maintain quality of imaging
- Create virtual unenhanced images
- Atherosclerotic plaque removal

Artefact reduction

- Reduce beam-hardening artefacts from metal and iodine
- Reduce photon starvation artefacts

Σ Summary

- Dual-energy CT utilises photoelectric effect
- Different materials attenuate individually along the beam energy spectrum - use this to separate out materials based on different attenuation at a high (140 kVp) and low (80 kVp) potentials

Techniques

- Dual-source: two x-ray tubes and two detectors
    - Simultaneous acquisition = faster, good overlap
    - Independently optimise tube-detector pair
    - Two scans = higher patient dose
    - Scatter from one system may be detected by other
- Single-source: single x-ray tube and two detectors
    - Consecutive
    - Sequential
    - Fast kVp switch
    - Twin-beam
- Detector-based spectral CT: single z-ray tube, single sandwich detector made of two layers to detect two energies

Applications

- Create virtual unenhanced images
- Use lower contrast dose
- Atherosclerotic plaque removal
- Virtual non-calcium images for MSK
- Detect silicon from breast implant leakage
- Better visualisation and characterisation of renal and hepatic lesions
- Artefact reduction

3.5 CT Image Quality

The image quality is mainly determined by 3 factors:

- Resolution
- Noise
- Contrast

Resolution

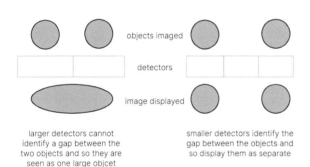

Figure 75   Resolution required to differentiate objects

Resolution is the measure of how far apart two objects must be before they can be seen as separate details in the image. For two objects to be seen as separate the detectors must be able to identify a gap between them.

Resolution is measured in line pairs per centimetre (lp/cm) i.e. the number of line pairs that can be imaged as separate structures within one centimetre.

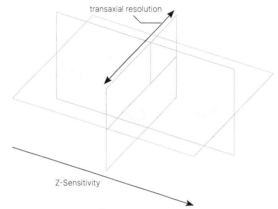

Figure 76   Types of resolution

There are two types of resolution in CT scanning:

- Transaxial resolution (7 lp/cm)
  - Axially across the patient
- Z-sensitivity (0.5 - 10 mm)
  - Along the length of the patient in the z-direction

Transaxial resolution

The minimum transaxial resolution is determined by the actual detector size, however it is often quoted as the "effective detector width" at the isocenter of the scanner (centre of the bore of the scanner). The "effective detector width" and the actual detector size are slightly different due to the divergence of the beam. The smaller the "effective detector width" the higher the resolution.

The transaxial resolution is affected by scanner (hardware) factors or scan and recon-struction parameters.

Scanner factors

1. Focal spot

▪ Size

Smaller focal spots give higher res-olution, but the max mA is limited to prevent damage to the anode.

There are usually two available focal spot sizes on CT scanners, for exam-ple:

• Fine = 0.7 mm

• Broad = 1.2 mm

▪ Properties

Flying focal spot: the position of the focal spot is rapidly altered in the transaxial plane and/or the Z-axis. Each focal spot position increases the number of projections sampled and improves spatial resolution. For ex-ample, if the position of the focal spot moves in the X-Y plane, then the in-plane resolution increases.

Focus-detector distance (FDD)

Focus-isocentre distance (FID)

2. Detector size

Smaller detectors give higher resolution but more detectors within an area also means more partitions (dead space) and a reduced overall detection efficiency.

3. Detector design properties

Quarter ray detector offset: the centre of the

detector array is offset from the centre of ro-tation by one quarter the width of an individ-ual detector. As the gantry rotates to 180° the centre of the detector array is now offset by half the width of a detector giving an inter-leaved sampling of the patient.

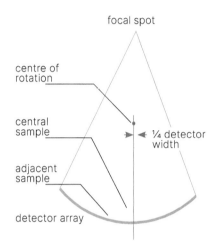

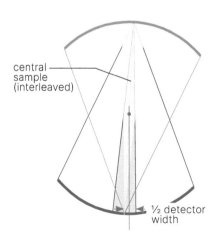

Figure 77   Quarter offset

Scan parameters

1. Number of projections

- Larger number of projections gives finer resolution (up to a point).

2. Reconstruction filter

- Higher resolution or "sharp" kernels (e.g. bone reconstruction) have better spatial resolution than soft kernels (e.g. soft tissue reconstruction).
- However, higher resolution kernels do not average out high spatial frequency signals and therefore produce more noise.

3. Pixel size

- The pixel size (d) in mm is give by the equation:

$$d = FOV/n$$

Where: FOV = field of view (mm)

n = image matrix size

- The highest spatial frequency that can be obtained (fmax) is called the Nyquist limit and is given by:

$$fmax = 1/2d$$

- From this equation you can see that the higher the pixel size, the lower the maximum spatial frequency.
- To improve spatial frequency we can:
  - Reduce the field of view (smaller FOV = smaller pixel size as seen in the first equation). We can do this retrospec-

tively by a targeted reconstruction of the original data into a small field of view.
  - Increase the matrix size (larger n = small pixel size as seen in the first equation)

Z-sensitivity

Z-sensitivity refers to the effective imaged slice width.

Factors affecting z-sensitivity

1. Detector slice thickness

- The wider (in the z-axis) the detector row, the lower the resolution

2. Overlapping samples

- Acquiring the data using overlapping slices can improve Z-sensitivity. This is achieved by using a low spiral pitch i.e. pitch <1.

3. Focal spot

- A fine focal spot improves the z-sensitivity

Importance of slice thickness

1. Noise

- The thinner the slice the better the resolution BUT the worse the noise

2. Partial volume effect

- Thicker slices increase the partial volume effects

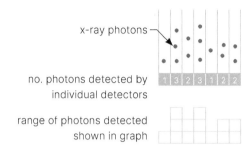

3. Isotropic scanning

- Thin slices allow isotropic scanning, i.e. the pixels in the axial and the z-axis are the same size (cubes). The advantages of this are:
  - Reduced partial volume effect
  - Better multi-planar reformatting
  - Improved volume rendering e.g. displaying 3D representations of the data (e.g. cardiac imaging, vascular imaging, CT colonography etc)

Noise

Even if we image a perfectly uniform object (e.g. a water filled object) there is still a variation in the Hounsfield units about a mean. This is due to noise. Noise degrades the image by degrading low contrast resolution and introducing uncertainty in the Hounsfield units of the images.

We can measure noise in any uniform region of the image e.g. with a water phantom. The standard deviation of the Hounsfield units in a selected region-of-interest gives the mean noise measurement.

There are three sources of noise:

1. Quantum noise
2. Electronic noise
3. Noise introduced by the reconstruction process e.g. backprojection.

Stochastic noise

Figure 78   Stochastic noise

This is the dominant source of noise in an image. Photon registration by the detectors is a stochastic process. The number of photons detected will vary randomly about a mean value and that variation is the noise. The noise in the final image is given by:

$$\text{Noise (standard deviation)} \propto 1/\sqrt{(\text{no. of photons})}$$

From this equation we can say that increasing the number of photons reduces the amount of noise and, therefore, anything that increases the number of photons (increases the photon flux) will reduce the noise. If we double the number of photons we will reduce the noise by $\sqrt{2}$ (i.e. increasing the number of photons by a factor of 4 will halve the noise).

Doubling the number of photons can be achieved by:

- Doubling the tube current (mA)
- Doubling the rotation time (s)
- Doubling the slice thickness (mm)

Increasing the tube kilovoltage (kV) also increases the photon flux but it is not directly proportional (output is approximately $\propto kV^2$).

Contrast

Factors influencing contrast:
- **Noise:** a higher noise will obscure any contrast between objects
- **Tube current:** a higher tube current reduces the noise in the image
- **Inherent tissue properties:** the difference in the linear attenuation coefficient of adjacent imaged objects will determine the contrast between those objects
- **Beam kilovoltage:** a higher beam energy will generally reduce the contrast between objects
- **Use of contrast media**

Summary

1) Resolution

Transaxial resolution
- Scanner factors
  - Focal spot size
  - Flying focal spot
  - Focus detector distance
  - Focus isocentre distance
  - Detector size
  - Quarter detector offset
- Scan parameters

- Number of projections
- Reconstruction filter
- Pixel size (d, mm) given by d = FOV/n (FOV=field of view, n=image matrix size)
- Highest spatial frequency (fmax) = 1/2d
- Not affected by:
  - Tube current
  - Tube kilovoltage

Z-sensitivity
- Equals effective slice thickness
- Affected by:
  - Detector slice thickness
  - Overlapping samples
  - Focal spot size
- Importance
  - Smaller the slice, greater the noise
  - Smaller the slice, the less the partial voluming artefact
  - Isotropic scanning enables better 3D reconstruction and MPR

2) Noise

Quantum noise
- Dominant source of noise
- Noise $\propto 1 / \sqrt{\text{no. of photons}}$
- Doubling the number of photons will decrease the noise by a factor of $\sqrt{2}$
- Doubling number of photons done by:
  - Doubling tube current (mA)
  - Doubling rotation time (s)
  - Doubling slice thickness (mm)

- Increasing the tube kilovoltage (kV) also increases the photon flux but it is not directly proportional

Others:
- Electronic noise in detection system
- Noise introduced by reconstruction e.g. backprojection

3) Contrast

Affected by:
- Noise: higher noise = worse contrast differentiation
- Tube current: lower tube current = more noise (see above)
- Inherent tissue properties: difference in linear attenuation coefficient of adjacent imaged objects determines contrast
- Beam kilovoltage: higher beam energy generally reduces contrast
- Use of contrast media: increases contrast between objects e.g. blood vessels and surrounding tissue

3.6 CT Artefacts

Causes of image artefacts can be grouped into a few categories:

- Physics based
- Patient properties
- Scanner based
- Helical and multislice artefacts

Physics Based

1) Beam hardening

An x-ray beam has photons of different energies that vary around a mean 'beam energy'. As the beam passes through a dense area the lower energy photons are more likely to be absorbed and the higher energy photons are more likely to remain. This results in a **higher mean beam energy**. This focally increased mean beam energy is interpreted as being due to it passing through a less attenuating material relative to the surroundings and so a lower Hounsfield unit is assigned and the image will be represented as more black.

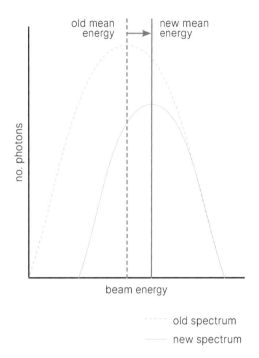

Figure 79 Beam hardening artefact

This is particularly common in the posterior fossa on a CT head scan due to the dense petrous bones.

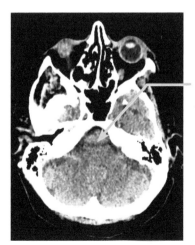

Figure 80 Beam hardening example

Cupping artefact

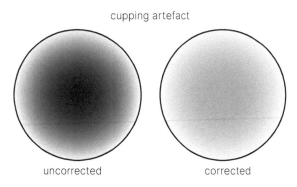

cupping artefact

uncorrected   corrected

Figure 81   Cupping artefact

This beam hardening artefact also produces another type of artefact called **the cupping artefact**. The centre of an object is usually the thickest and, therefore, the beam will become harder in the centre than at the periphery and is assigned lower Hounsfield units. This can be corrected with a 'beam hardening correction' algorithm.

Solutions to beam hardening

- **Pre-patient filter:** This absorbs the soft x-rays and minimises the beam hardening artefact
- **Bow-tie filter:** Pre-harden the x-ray beam

2) Partial volume artefact

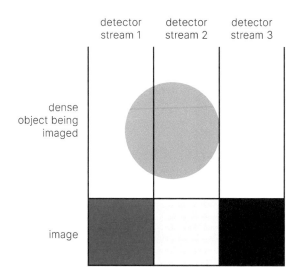

detector stream 1   detector stream 2   detector stream 3

dense object being imaged

image

Figure 82   Partial volume artefact

If a dense object only partially protrudes into a detector stream the attenuation is averaged with its surroundings and it will be assigned a lower Hounsfield unit. In the image above, the dense circle lies on a less dense background. The object fills detector stream 2 resulting in a very high attenuation (white). In detector stream 3 none of the dense object is imaged and so the attenuation is low (black). In detector stream 1 the object is only partially imaged and so the attenuation is an average between the dense object and the less dense background.

N.B. partial voluming will only ever **reduce** the apparent attenuation of an object, it will never **increase** the apparent attenuation.

3) Incomplete projection

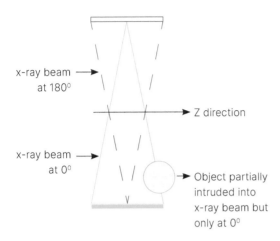

x-ray beam →
at 180⁰

→ Z direction

x-ray beam →
at 0⁰

→ Object partially
intruded into
x-ray beam but
only at 0⁰

Figure 83   Streak artefact

An object may protrude into the slice in one projection but not in the opposing projection, especially at the periphery of the image where the beam is more divergent. If this happens, a variant of partial voluming artefact occurs in which the object appears streaked due to the inconsistencies produced during imaging.

These streak artefacts can be caused, for example, when a patient's arms are by their side and are imaged in some projections but not others.

Solution
▪ Smaller slice thickness

4) Photon starvation

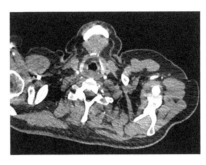

There are white lines across the shoulders on this CT image from side to side. This is the noise from photom starvation

Figure 84   Photon starvation example

This is another cause of streak artefacts. In projections that have to travel through more material, e.g. across the shoulders, as the x-ray beam travels through more x-ray photons are absorbed and removed from the beam. This results in a smaller proportion of signal reaching the detector and, therefore, a larger proportion of noise. The streaks are due to the increased noise which is why they occur in the direction of the widest part of the object being scanned.

Solutions
▪ **Adaptive filtering:** the regions in which the attenuation exceeds a specified level are smoothed before undergoing back-projection.

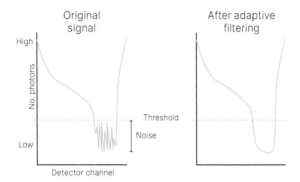

Figure 85 Adaptive filtering

- **mA modulation:** the tube current (mA) can be varied with the gantry rotation. HIgher mA's (greater signal) are used for the more attenuating projections to reduce the effect of photon starvation. The mA required can either be calculated in advance from the scout view or during the scan from the feedback system of the detector.

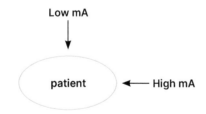

Figure 86 Current modulation

Patient Properties

1) Metallic artefacts

The metal produces a beam-hardening and photon starvation artefact. This can also happen with other high attenuation materials such as IV contrast.

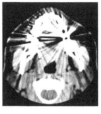 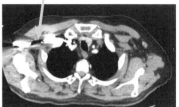

Figure 87 Metal artefact example

2) Patient motion

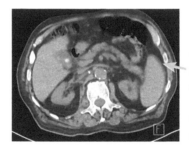

Figure 88 Motion artefact example

Motion artefact can be caused by:
- Patient swallowing
- Breathing
- Pulsatility of heart and vessels
- Patient moving

If a patient or structure moves as the gantry rotates the object will be detected as being in several positions and represented in the image as such.

Solutions
- Scan parameters

- Shorten scan time
- Spiral scanning
- ECG gating: this can be used pro-spectively to trigger image acquisition during a specific point on the ECG when heart motion is lowest, or retro-spectively by reconstructing acquired data from specific ECG phases
- Patient parameters
  - Breath hold
  - Ensure comfortable patient position
  - Tell patient to stay still and give clear instructions

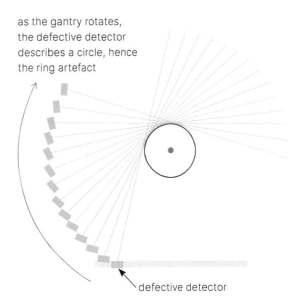

as the gantry rotates, the defective detector describes a circle, hence the ring artefact

defective detector

Figure 89   Ring artefact

3) Incomplete projections

If there are objects lying outside the field of view, especially high attenuation objects such as the arms, this will create streak artefacts within the imaged area as the arms will be detected in some projections and not others leading to inconsistencies in the data.

Scanner Based

1) Ring artefact

If there is a faulty detector and the detectors do not have the same gain relative to each other (they are operating at different base-lines) then as the gantry rotates around the patient this detector will outline a circle. On back-projection this will cause a **ring artefact**.

Spiral and Multislice Scanning Artefacts

1) Helical artefacts

In spiral scanning, as the gantry rotates it is also moving in the z-axis. This means that a row of detectors is moving in a spiral path. This can cause artefactual representation of structures that are changing in shape or po-sition in the z-axis as they will be in different positions for different projections used in the reconstruction of the image. Nowadays this artefact is rare as scanners have a large num-ber of detectors and pitch <1.

Worsened by:
- Increasing pitch
- Increased contrast between object and surrounding structures

2) Cone beam artefact

Fan Beam

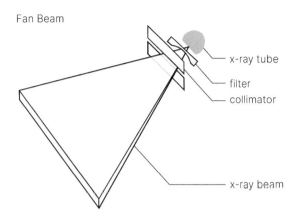

Cone Beam

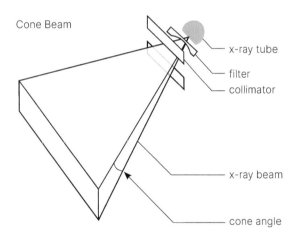

Figure 90   Comparison of fan beam and cone beam

This is a particular artefact caused by multislice scanners. As the section scanned increases per rotation, a wider collimation is used. Because of this the x-ray beam becomes cone-shaped instead of fan-shaped and the area imaged by each detector as it rotates around the patient is a volume instead of a flat plane. The resulting artefact is similar to the partial volume artefact for off-centre objects. This is particularly pronounced at the edges of the image. With modern scanners cone beam reconstruction algorithms correct this artefact.

The cone beam effect is assessed with a **Capthan test phantom.**

Solution
▪ Reconstruction algorithm minimises cone beam artefacts

Summary

1) Physics based

Beam hardening
▪ Dense objects remove more lower energy photons from the x-ray beam leaving a higher average energy beam. A higher average energy of incident beam is interpreted as having passed through a structure that causes less attenuation of the beam and represented as such on the image (i.e. black bands)
▪ **Cupping**: variation of beam hardening that occurs in spherical objects. Corrected with a beam hardening correction algorithm
▪ Solutions:
   ◦ Pre-patient filter to absorb soft x-rays
   ◦ Bow-tie filter to equalise the attenuation across the patient profile

Partial volume artefact
▪ If object is smaller than slice thickness its attenuation will be averaged within the

slice resulting in a displayed lower attenuation of the object
- **Incomplete projection:** variation of partial volume artefact in which an object is present in the x-ray beam in some projections and not others causing streak artefact
- Solutions:
  - Thinner slices

2) Patient properties

Metallic artefact
- Analogous to beam hardening artefact caused by high density structures such as metal or iodinated contrast.
- Solutions:
  - Same as for beam hardening
  - Avoid metal in imaged region

Movement artefact
- Solutions:
  - Breath hold
  - ECG gating with prospective or retrospective image formation
  - Ensure patient in comfortable position
  - Tell patient to stay still and give clear instructions
  - Short scan time
  - Spiral scanning

3) Scanner based

- **Ring artefact:** caused by a faulty detector element or incorrect relative gain setting

4) Spiral and multislice based

- **Helical artefacts:** As gantry rotates it is moving in the z-axis. Any object that changes in position or size along the z-axis may be distorted as they will be in different positions for different projections
- **Cone beam artefact:** Due to wider collimation, the beam has a volume and becomes cone-shaped. A similar artefact to partial voluming occurs for off-centre objects in the detector field. The artefact is worse for objects at the edges of the beam.

3.7   CT Dose

Units of Dose

We can think of the different dose measurements as a stepwise progression, each time adding an additional variable into the equation.

1) CT Dose Index (CTDI)

First, we measure the dose to the detectors from a single gantry rotation to give us the **CTDI**.

CT dose index

Definition	Dose to the phantom from single gantry rotation
Units	mGy
Affected by	Collimator Focus-isocentre distance

2) Weighted CTDI (CTDI$_w$)

The dose is not equal across the scan plane. It is higher in the periphery than in the centre. We need to adjust for this by making the average periphery dose make up 2/3 of the dose to give us the **weighted CTDI**.

There are separate calculations for imaging the head, body and paediatric patients. In adults we use a head phantom (16 cm) and a body phantom (32 cm) with dosimeters placed at the periphery and centre in order to calculate the weighted average of doses.

Weighted CTDI

Definition	Adjusted for spatial variation of dose
Equation	$CTDI_w = 1/3\ CTDI_{centre} + 2/3\ CTDI_{periphery}$
Units	mGy

3) Volume CTDI (CTDI$_{vol}$)

We don't scan single slices. The concentration of the dose along a patient is determined by the **pitch**. The higher the pitch, the larger the gaps between slices and the lower the dose. Taking into account the pitch gives us the **volume CTDI**.

Volume CTDI

Definition	Accounts for effect of pitch. Higher pitch = lower dose as less overlapping. However, many manufacturers autocompensate for changes in pitch by adjusting mA to keep the noise and dose constant.
Equation	$CTDI_{vol} = CTDI_w\ /\ pitch$
Units	mGy

4) Dose length product (DLP)

Now we know the CDTI$_{vol}$, we multiply this by the distance along the patient we have scanned to give us the **dose length product**. It is proportional to the radiation risk to the patient.

Dose length product

Definition	Total dose to phantom / patient along the distance scanned
Equation	DLP = CTDI$_{vol}$ x distance scanned
Units	mGy*cm

5) Effective dose (E)

We now have the total dose along the patient. But radiation does not affect all organs equally. Each organ has a **sensitivity** to radiation that needs to be taken into account. We display this as the **effective dose**.

Effective dose

Definition	Physical effect of total dose on patient determined by the susceptibility of imaged area to radiation
Equation	In the latest ICRP103 guideline the equation used to calculate effective dose is: $E = \Sigma T\ (W_T) \times \Sigma R\ (W_R D_{T,R})$ or $E = \Sigma\ W_T H_T$ Key: H_T or $W_T D_{T,R}$ is the equivalent dose in a tissue or organ (T) W_T is the tissue weighting factor
Units	Millisieverts (mSv) or J.kg^{-1} - note that the units have changed as this is the effective dose to patients.

\

Factors Affecting Dose

- **Tube current**
  - Doubling mA = doubling of CTDI, DLP and E
- **Rotation time**
  - Doubling rotation time = doubling of CTDI, DLP and E
- **Pitch**
  - Doubling pitch = halving of CTDI, DLP and E
- **kVp**
  - Dose is approximately $\propto$ kVp^2 i.e. doubling the kVp will increase the dose by a factor of 4 (approximately).

Summary

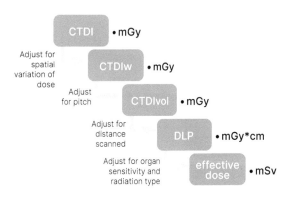

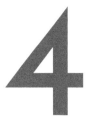

Ultrasound imaging makes use of sound waves at frequencies beyond the range of human hearing. These waves pass through tissues, get reflected, and the returning wave (echo) is detected and forms the image. In B-mode imaging, the most common imaging used in medicine, the intensity of the returning wave is represented as a level of brightness on the monitor to give a 2D cross-sectional image on the monitor.

This chapter focuses on the physics, production and manipulation of sound by the ultrasound machine to create an image. It also covers the artefacts created during imaging.

4.1	Properties of Sound	115
4.2	Ultrasound Machine	119
4.3	Producing an Ultrasound Beam	123
4.4	Image Properties	127
4.5	Doppler	130
4.6	US Artefacts	134

4.1   Properties of Sound

Sound waves are very different from electro-magnetic (EM) radiation.

Sound waves	X-rays
Mechanical energy	EM radiation
Requires a medium	Can travel in a vacuum
Longitudinal wave: particles in the medium move back and forth parallel to the direction the wave is travelling	Transverse wave: electric and magnetic component oscillating at right angles to each other, and to the direction of propagation
Variable velocity	Constant velocity

Anatomy of a Sound Wave

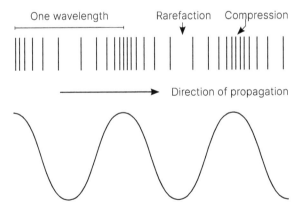

Figure 91   Anatomy of a sound wave

As the sound wave passes through material the particles vibrate back and forth. In some areas the particles are close together (compression) and in others they are further apart (rarefaction). A sound wave can also be represented sinusoidally with the peaks and troughs of the wave corresponding to the areas of maximum compression and rarefaction.

1) Frequency

The audible range of sound waves for humans is 20 to 20,000 Hz. 1 Hz is 1 wavelength per second. Medical ultrasound uses frequencies of **2-18 MHz** (1 MHz = 1 million Hz) i.e. above the range of human hearing..

2) Velocity

The velocity of a sound wave is dependent on, and constant for, the material through which the wave is passing.

$$c = \sqrt{(k / \rho)}$$

Where: c = speed
k = rigidity
ρ = density

From the above equation, the speed of the sound wave increases with increasing rigidity and decreasing density. It travels the slowest in air as the material is so compressible that a lot of energy is lost between the particles. The important number to learn is that for soft tissues the speed is around 1540 m/s. Ultrasound machines are calibrated to this speed to give the best images of soft tissues.

Material	Speed of sound (m/s)
Air	330
Water	1480
Tissue	1540
Bone	4080

3) Wavelength

One wavelength is the distance between two identical points in the wave cycle i.e. the distance between the point of peak compression and the next peak compression. The **wavelength** is inversely proportional to the **frequency** and proportional to the **velocity** of the sound wave. In ultrasound imaging, however, the frequency is set by the transducer so it is mainly the velocity that affects the wavelength.

$$c = f \, l$$

Where: c = velocity

f = frequency

l = wavelength

4) Intensity

The intensity of a sound wave is measured in watts per metre^2 (w/m^2). The decibel scale is used to represent the ratio of two intensities.

$$\text{dB ratio} = 10 \log^{10} (I_1 / I_2)$$

Where: I_1 = intensity one

I_2 = intensity two

If the attenuation coefficient is 1 dB/cm, after travelling through 10 cm of tissue, the intensity will be reduced by 10 dB or a factor of 10. After 20 cm it would be reduced by 20 dB or a factor of 100

Interaction with Tissue

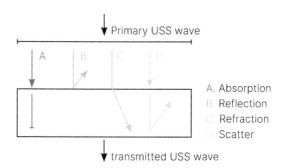

Figure 92   Interaction of sound waves with tissues

An ultrasound beam interacts with tissue and is attenuated via four mechanisms:

1. Absorption
2. Reflection
3. Refraction
4. Scatter

1) Absorption

This is the main cause of attenuation. Energy is transferred to the material it is traveling through as heat. The energy of the ultra-sound wave decreases exponentially. Higher frequencies are absorbed more rapidly and, therefore, decrease in intensity and are absorbed more quickly.

2) Reflection

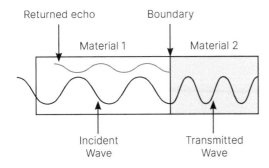

Figure 93   Echo of an ultrasound

This occurs at the interface/tissue boundaries. The amount of reflection depends on the difference between the **acoustic impedance (Z)** of the tissues at an interface **(acoustic impedance mismatch)**. This is one reason gel is used in ultrasound, to reduce the acoustic impedance mismatch between the transducer and the skin and to minimise the amount of trapped air between the transducer and the skin. This minimises reflection of the sound wave. At a soft tissue-air interface, over 99% of the echo is reflected.

The acoustic impedance is a measure of how easily material allows sound waves to pass through, the higher the impedance mismatch, the more of the wave that is reflected:

>Acoustic impedance (Z) (kg m^{-2} s^{-1}) = density x speed of sound in that material

Reflection coefficient (R) = $(Z_2 - Z_1)^2 / (Z_2 + Z_1)^2$

Bone	Highest Z
Liver	
Blood	
Water	
Fat	
Gas	Lowest Z

- Good transmitters:
  - Small light molecules as they don't need as much energy to move them
  - Material with stiff bonds as energy travels quicker through stiffer bonds
- Poor transmitters:
  - Large dense molecules with weak bonds

3) Refraction

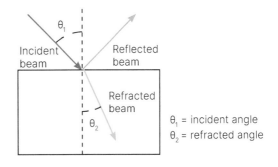

θ_1 = incident angle
θ_2 = refracted angle

Figure 94   Refraction and reflection of a beam

When an ultrasound wave crosses an interface between two tissue some of the beam is reflected, the rest passes into the material. As the beam passes into the second material, the velocity changes. This causes refraction, or bending, of the ultrasound wave. The angle of refraction depends on the velocity change of the wave after it has crossed the interface.

4) Scatter

When a sound wave interacts with an object smaller than a wavelength and most of the beam doesn't interact with it the sound wave is scattered. This is in contrast to when objects are larger than the wavelength In which case they are reflected.

Scatter increases when:
- Decreased size of the object causing scatter
- Increased acoustic impedance mismatch

Summary

1) Anatomy of a sound wave

- Frequency
  - The range of sound audible by humans is 20-20,000 Hz
  - Medical imaging uses ultrasound waves of 2-18 MHz
- Velocity
  - Velocity = $\sqrt{}$ (rigidity / density)
  - Velocity faster in bone than air
  - 1540 m/s in most soft tissues
- Wavelength
  - Velocity = frequency x wavelength
  - Wavelength inversely proportional to frequency and proportional to velocity. Frequency set by transducer.
- Intensity
  - Measured in watts/m^2
  - Also measured as the attenuation of sound in decibels (dB) which is the log ratio between two intensities

2) Interaction with matter

Occurs via three mechanisms:
- Absorption: main mechanism. More quickly absorbed in higher frequencies
- Reflection: more reflection when higher impedance mismatch. At a soft tissue-air interface, over 99% of the wave is reflected
- Refraction: change in velocity when beam crosses an interface causing change in angle
- Scatter: when particle smaller than a wavelength beam scattered in all directions

4.2   Ultrasound Machine

Modes

1) A-Mode (A for Amplitude)

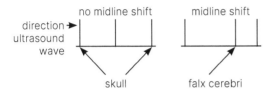

Figure 95   A mode of ultrasound

One beam of ultrasound is passed through the material and the returning echoes are recorded giving a 1D representation of the structures the beam passes through. A-mode was the first use of medical ultrasound and was used to show midline shift in the brain. An ultrasound beam was passed through the skull and the bones and falx would return the echoes showing their position. Now, it is mainly used in ophthalmology to investigate retinal detachment etc.

2) B-Mode (B for Brightness)

This is now the main mode of ultrasound used. The echoes returned are shown on screen in a grey-scale corresponding to their intensity. The structures are shown as a 2D image on screen.

3) M-Mode (M for Motion)

Ultrasound waves are released in quick succession in A or B-mode and recorded. This creates an image analogous to a video recording.

As organ boundaries reflecting the sound waves move, the velocity can be calculated e.g. heart valves.

4) Doppler

Uses the Doppler effect to measure flow e.g. blood flow. As a sound wave hits a moving object the returning sound wave changes in frequency. If the object is moving towards the transducer the frequency increases, if the object is moving away from the transducer the frequency decreases. Doppler can be pulsed or continuous.

B-Mode Transducer

1) Basics

- 100 or more A-lines are fired sequentially
- These are reflected from the tissue interfaces
- The amplitude of the returning waves are received and converted into brightness
- An image is built up line-by-line forming a cross-sectional image

2) Transducer

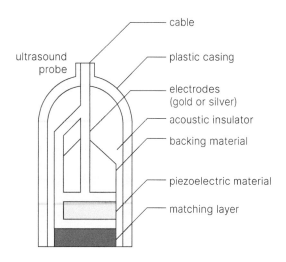

Figure 96   Ultrasound transducer

The transducer converts mechanical energy into electrical energy and vice versa. It acts as both a transmitter and a receiver of sound.

Acoustic Insulator: stops the transducer vibrating in the hand.

Backing Material: stops vibrations reverberating back into the piezoelectric material. It determines the length of the ultrasound pulse by determining how much it is dampened (Q value, see chapter 4.3 - Producing an Ultrasound Beam).

Piezoelectric Material: material that forms ultrasounds and receives echoes. It is ½ wavelength thick and is usually composed of 256 crystals.

Matching Layer: always ¼ wavelength thick to reduce wavelength impedance difference.

Safety

The advantages of ultrasound imaging are:
- No radiation exposure
- Non-invasive
- Fast
- Inexpensive
- Real-time imaging
- Can measure velocity e.g. of blood
- Cross-sectional imaging

There are also disadvantages to ultrasound:
- Can't image through bone or gas
- Very dependent on operator skill

Although ultrasound is generally safe and there has been no confirmed evidence of damage from diagnostic ultrasound exposure, there are some theoretical risks. There are a few values that must be monitored and kept within certain limits to reduce the likelihood of these risks.
- Time-averaged intensity <100 mWcm^{-2}
- Total sound energy <50 Jcm^{-2}
- Thermal index
- Mechanical index

1) Thermal Index (TI)

The TI measures the ability of the ultrasound to heat up the local tissue.

TI = power emitted / that required to increase temperature by 1°c

An index of <0.5 is below the threshold level for any effect and considered safe. As the TI increases the scanning time should be decreased in proportion e.g. with a TI of 3 a patient may be scanned for 10 min. If the patient has a fever, the threshold for complications is lower and the scanning time should be shortened e.g. with TI of 3 and a patient with a temperature of 39°c scanning for even less than 1 min would not be safe.

Sensitive tissues that are more susceptible to thermal damage are:
- An embryo less than eight weeks after conception
- The head, brain or spine of any fetus or neonate
- The eye (in a subject of any age).

2) Mechanical Index (MI)

The MI is the measure of the maximum amplitude of the pressure pulse and indicates the risk of cavitation.

$$MI = peak\ negative\ pressure\ /\ \sqrt{(ultrasound\ frequency)}$$

The British Medical Ultrasound Society (BMUS) states that general diagnostic ultrasound and obstetric ultrasound must have an MI <0.7, especially with the use of contrast agents which theoretically increase the cavitation risk with higher MIs. The MI in general neonatal imaging should be <0.5.

3) Complications of ultrasound

- **Local heating**
- **Cavitation:** The pressure changes cause microbubbles in a liquid to expand then collapse. There is an increased risk of cavitation in:
  - Gas-containing structures (e.g. bowel, lung)
  - Low frequency pulses (i.e. longer wavelengths)
  - Higher power or intensity of pulses
  - Use of ultrasound contrast agent.
- **Mechanical damage** to cell membranes

Summary

1) Modes

- A-Mode - (amplitude) 1D representation of structures
- B-Mode - (brightness) most commonly used form of diagnostic ultrasound
- M-Mode - (motion) used in cardiac imaging
- Doppler - measures flow and velocity

2) Transducer

- Backing material: determines pulse length via Q-value
- Piezoelectric crystals: produce and receive ultrasound beam. ½ wavelength

thick
- Matching layer: reduces impedance difference. ¼ wavelength thick

3) Safety

- Time-averaged intensity < 100 mWcm^{-2}
- Total sound energy < 50 Jcm^{-2}
- Thermal index
    - Indicates risk of local heating
    - TI 0 - 1.0 safe
    - Decreased threshold in: febrile patients, fetal scanning, eye
    - Should never use TI > 3 in fetal scanning
- Mechanical index
    - Indicates risk of cavitation
    - MI < 0.7 for general use
    - MI < 0.5 for fetal scanning
    - MI > 0.7 should never be used with ultrasound contrast agents
- Complications
    - Local heating, cavitation, mechanical damage

4.3   Producing an Ultrasound Beam

Piezoelectric Effect

A transducer with piezoelectric crystals is used to produce the ultrasound beam. This is a material in which mechanical energy is converted into electrical energy and vice versa. This means that transmitting an electric voltage through the material will cause it to vibrate, producing a sound wave. Similarly, the returning echo sound wave vibrates the crystals producing an electric voltage that can be measured. In this way, the material acts as a receiver and a transmitter. The intensity of the sound wave, or the pressure changes, is proportional to the amount of voltage. The system can, therefore, represent the intensity of the returning echoes as points of brightness (B-mode imaging) based on the voltage produced.

cross in the same phase, they combine and are reinforced (constructive interference). If, however, they are in different phases they cancel each other out (destructive interference).

A transducer produces its largest output when the frequency produces a wavelength equal to 2x the thickness of the piezoelectric disc. This is because as the material pulses backwards and forwards it reinforces the waves due to them being exactly in-phase. Therefore, the crystals are cut to half the thickness of the desired wavelength.

*** Thickness of piezoelectric disc = 1/2 λ (desired wavelength) ***

1) Natural / resonant frequency

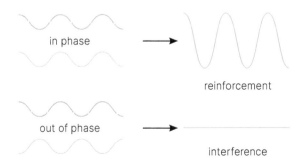

in phase

reinforcement

out of phase

interference

Figure 97   Phase of ultrasound wave

If two sound waves of the same wavelength

2) Pulse duration

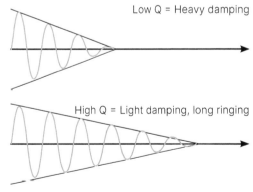

Low Q = Heavy damping

High Q = Light damping, long ringing

Figure 98   Q value and pulse duration

Once the transducer is pushed it continues to vibrate for a short time with exponentially decreasing intensity **(damping)**. The mechanical coefficient (Q value) reflects how quickly the signal is dampened.

Materials with a higher Q-value vibrate for a long time i.e. have a light dampening effect, and the pulse persists for a longer time. Materials with a low Q-value dampen the vibration quickly and the pulse lasts for a shorter time.

3) Pulse Repetition Frequency (PRF)

The scan line density is the number of beams sent out by the transducer to sample the patient's tissues per frame.

The typical number is 100 lines per frame. To allow adequate real-time image a sufficiently large number of frames must be scanned per second. The rate at which these frames are repeated is measured by the pulse repetition frequency (PRF). It depends upon the velocity of sound (which is assumed to be ~1500 m/s), the depth of the structure being imaged and the number of pulses sent out per frame.

PRF = frame rate x lines per frame

e.g. 30 frames per second each of 100 lines per frame requires a PRF of 3 kHz

Longer PRF caused by:
- Deeper structures being imaged (the longer it takes to go and come back, the longer the listen phase of the pulse has to be)

- More lines per frame

4) Depth of view

In each pulse the beam has to be transmitted, reach the structure to be imaged, and the echo returned to the transducer before the next pulse can be generated. The time taken to reach a structure, the distance the beam travels and the speed of the beam are related to each other by the equation below.

Distance = time x velocity x 0.5

(divide by 2 for journey there and back)

Each pulse has to go to the deepest tissue then return to the transducer before the next pulse is generated. The depth of tissues that can be imaged with a particular PRF can be calculated by the equation below:

Depth of view = 0.5 x sound velocity / PRF

Transducer Array

1) Single Transducer

When a single transducer produces a beam it starts off as a parallel beam (near field). This is the most useful part of the beam. Then, the beam diverges (far field). The length of this near field depends on the width of the transducer. The wider the transducer the longer the near field.

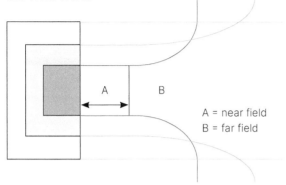

Figure 99 Single transducer near field

$$\text{Near field distance} = D^2 / 4\lambda$$

Where: D = diameter of transducer
          λ = wavelength

To get as long a near field distance as possible we would have to make the transducer wider. However, the resolution will be reduced and the width of the whole transducer array will be much larger. To overcome this, a stepped linear array is used.

2) Stepped linear array

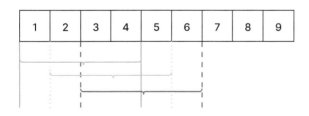

Figure 100 Stepped linear array

Many small transducers are placed next to each other. They are then activated as a group to widen the beam and produce a longer near field distance. The initial transducer is then inactivated and the next transducer activated, moving the beam along. In this way many more wide beams can be produced in a smaller space than could be produced with wide transducers activated individually.

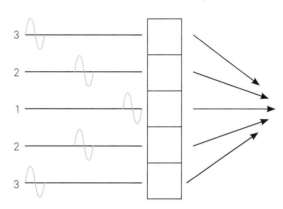

Figure 101 Focusing a beam

This linear array can also be used to focus the beam electronically. The outermost transducers are activated first, then the two inner, then the innermost etc. In this way the transmitted beam is focused to a specific point. The order in which transducers receive echoes can also be focused to preferentially receive signals from a particular depth. This is what happens when the focus is set on the ultrasound machine.

Summary

- Piezoelectric effect is a property of the transducer crystals. An electric current produces movement and vice versa.

- Thickness of piezoelectric crystal = 1/2 x desired λ
- Mechanical coefficient (Q value) of backing material
  - High Q value = low dampening, long pulse
  - Low Q value = heavy dampening, short pulse
- Pulse repetition frequency (PRF) = frame rate x lines per frame
- Distance travelled by beam = time x velocity x 0.5
- Depth of view = 0.5 x sound velocity / PRF
- Near field distance = (diameter of transducer)^2 / 4λ
- Stepped linear array increases near field distance and can be used to electronically focus the beam

4.4 Image Properties

Spatial Resolution

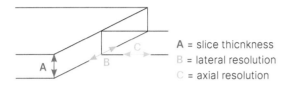

A = slice thicnkness
B = lateral resolution
C = axial resolution

Figure 102 Resolution of a beam

1) Axial resolution

The ability to differentiate between two objects in the axial plane, i.e. along the path of the ultrasound beam, depends on the **length of the ultrasound pulse** and the **wavelength**. The resolution is increased by:
- Low Q value of backing material (shorter pulse length)
- Shorter wavelength i.e. increased frequency

2) Lateral resolution

The lateral resolution is measured perpendicular to the direction of the ultrasound beam and depends on the beam width which, in turn, depends on the diameter of the PZT crystals and the focusing. To differentiate between two objects, you need at least three beams to interact, one on each object and then one in the space between the two objects. Lateral resolution is always worse than axial resolution and it corresponds to ~1/3 of the transducer diameter.

$$Beam\ width = focal\ length\ x\ \lambda / D$$

Where: λ = wavelength
D = diameter

3) Slice thickness

The higher the frequency the smaller the slice thickness. It is usually larger than the beam width. For standard 2D transducers the slice thickness is fixed.

Temporal Resolution

This is the ability of the system to display events occurring at different times as separate images. It is measured in frames per second. It is reduced by:
- Greater number of focal zones
- Having doppler on
- Deeper object (echo takes longer to reach object and return)
- Large sector width (more space to scan)

Each pulse of a transmitter contains a transmit (during which the ultrasound wave is produced) and a receive (during which the transducer "listens" for the returning echo) phase. The **pulse repetition frequency (PRF)** is the number of pulses of ultrasound sent out by the transducer per second. It depends on the velocity of sound and the depth of the tissue being imaged - the deeper the tissue, the longer the transducer has to wait for the echoes to come back i.e. lower PRF.

Harmonics

At higher intensities the speed of sound is slightly faster in the high pressure (compression) parts than in the low pressure (rarefaction) which skews the normal sinusoidal wave.

- The leading edge of the sinusoidal wave becomes deeper
- Effect increases the deeper the wave travels
- This degrades the image at depth

When you perform a Fourier analysis of the returning wave, the frequencies returned are **harmonic** i.e. if a 2 MHz pulse is sent out, the harmonic frequencies returned are 4 MHz, 6 MHz and 8 MHz etc.

When turning on the harmonics function on the ultrasound machine an electronic filter or pulse inversion technique ensures the fundamental frequency is not returned and the harmonic frequencies are used to build up the picture.

1) Advantages

- Higher frequencies generated at the tissue interface have less distance to travel (only travel one way, not there and back)
- Contains fewer reverberation artefacts. The harmonics used to develop the picture are developed at deeper structures whereas reverberation comes from shallow structures.
- Better resolution at deeper structures

2) When to use it

- **Cardiac work:** reduces reverberation from ribs. Reduces movement artefacts from tachycardia and respiration.
- **Fluid-filled structures:** reduces reverberation artefacts. Improves contrast.
- Improved edge enhancement
- Obese patients
- **Carotid arteries:** measuring wall thickness and atheroma

3) Limitations

- Not so useful in superficial structures
- Effects lost in very deep structures
- Safety: need high power USS

Compound Imaging

This utilises a phenomenon known as "beam steering" in which the angle of the ultrasound beam is altered. In compound imaging the beam is transmitted at up to 9 different angles per sweep. The same object is imaged at different angles. This means that some beams will reach behind the object and return echoes.

- **Advantages:** useful when examining small parts and superficial structures.
- **Disadvantages:** takes away useful artefacts (acoustic shadow). Reduces frame rate.

- Compound imaging useful for small/superficial structures but removes acoustic shadow

Summary

- Axial resolution improved by:
  - Shorter wavelength (higher frequency)
  - Shorter length of pulse (lower Q-value of backing material)
- Lateral resolution improved by:
  - Smaller beam width
- Temporal resolution worsened by:
  - Smaller PRF
  - Deeper structures
  - More focal zones
  - Doppler
  - Larger sector width
- Harmonics used in obese patients and to improve movement/reverberation artefacts

4.5 Doppler

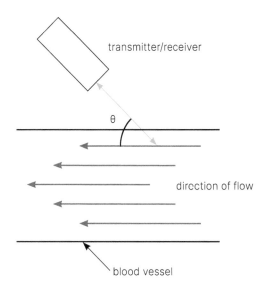

transmitter/receiver

θ

dircetion of flow

blood vessel

Figure 103 Doppler

When sound is reflected from a moving object, such as blood cells, the returned echoes are at a different frequency to that of the original sound source and the amount of change in the frequency is proportional to the velocity of the interface.

- If the object is moving away from the source, the frequency decreases.
- If the object is moving towards the source, the frequency increases.

As the angle between the transmitter and the interface (insonation angle) nears 90° the accuracy of the estimation of the velocity of the interface decreases. In general use, **an insonation angle of less than 60°** is used to give accurate estimates of velocity.

Continuous Wave Doppler

These are usually dedicated handheld devices (e.g. ABPIs, cardiotopograms for fetal heartwave). The Doppler effect is emitted as an audible sound due to the Doppler shift being in the audible sound frequency range: the higher the pitch the greater the velocity; the harsher the sound the more turbulent the flow. As they transmit (and, therefore, receive) continuously, they have to contain two separate transmit and receive elements.

Advantages
- Cheap
- Easy to use
- Sensitive to flow

Disadvantages
- Can't measure velocity
- Insonate all vessels in the beam path until the beam is attenuated. This means that as arteries and veins usually lie close together the output often combines arterial and venous signals.
- Can't determine depth

Pulsed Wave Doppler

In pulsed wave Doppler, the same elements

are used for transmitting and receiving and brief pulses of ultrasound energy are emitted. Range gating is used to only accept echoes returning from a specific depth. Duplex involves Doppler imaging overlayed over B-mode imaging.

There are three types of pulsed wave Doppler used in ultrasound machines:

- Colour
- Power
- Spectral

1) Colour doppler

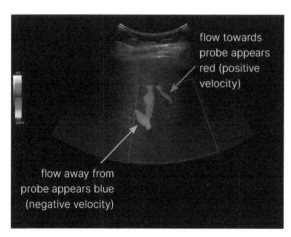

Figure 104 Doppler example

In colour Doppler the **sampling volume** is set and the mean and variance of the velocity of the moving structures calculated. This velocity is then represented by a scale of arbitrary colours ranging from minus (moving away from the transducer) to zero (no calculated velocity) to plus (moving towards transducer). The pulse frame rate affects the real-time colour Doppler measurement. A lower frame rate results in a stuttering colour Doppler e.g. using a larger Doppler sampling box which requires more Doppler pulses and, therefore, lowers the frame rate.

2) Power doppler

Power Doppler images map the **amplitude only** of the Doppler signal without any indication of the velocity. All movement, regardless of phase, contributes to the amplitude. This means that power Doppler emphasises the quantity of blood flow.

Advantages
- Less dependent on insonation angle
- Can show very low flow rates
- Not subject to aliasing

Disadvantages
- No indication of flow direction
- Tissue motion creates artefacts

3) Spectral doppler

Spectral Doppler shows the range of Doppler frequencies returned over time and displayed in a **sonogram**.

Differences in vessel wall resistance produce different spectral traces. The characteristics of the vessel walls can be represented numerically as the **Resistive Index (RI)** and the

Pulsatility Index (PI).

RI = (peak systolic frequency - end diastolic
frequency) /
peak systolic frequency

PI = (peak systolic frequency - minimum
frequency) /
time averaged maximum frequency

High resistance vessel
Highly pulsatile with sharp upstroke and narrow range of velocities e.g. peripheral vessels such as femoral artery and aorta.

Low resistance artery
Low pulsatility with large range of velocities e.g. in vessels supplying vital organs that need flow even during diastole such as renal artery, internal carotid artery.

Normal RI = 0.6 - 0.7

Abnormal RI = 0.8 - 1.0

Artefacts

1) Aliasing

The Nyquist limit states that the sampling frequency must be greater than twice the highest frequency of the input signal in order to be able to accurately represent the image.

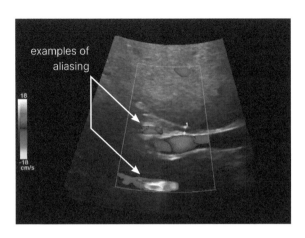

Figure 105 Aliasing in doppler

Nyquist limit = PRF / 2

If the velocity of the flow is greater than the Nyquist limit, the Doppler shift exceeds the scale and "wrap-around" occurs.

2) Spectral broadening

Blood flowing closer the inside of the vessel wall is slower than flow in the middle of the vessel. This large range of frequencies in a particular moment in time produces a widening of the spectral graph and different colours in colour Doppler. This also occurs with turbulent flow (e.g. stenotic vessels) as the turbulence creates flow of different velocities and directions.

3) Doppler angle

Flow velocity estimation requires the flow to be as parellel to the direction of the ultrasound beam as possible. If it is perpendicular, i.e. traveling across the beam, flow is difficult to detect. The angle of insonation should be less than 60° at all times to allow the most accurate estimation of velocity.

4) Wall filters

An electronic filter is applied to the returning data to eliminate low frequency signals as these are usually produced by low velocity structures such as vessel walls. If the filter is inappropriately applied the real signals from low velocity blood flow are eliminated.

Summary

1) Doppler

Doppler effect.
- Flow moving away = decrease in returning frequency
- Flow moving towards = increase in returning frequency

Continuous wave Doppler
- Separate transmit and receive elements for continuous measurement of flow requiring dedicated probe

- Can't differentiate between two structures
- Can't determine depth

Pulsed wave Doppler
- Can display on top of B-mode (called duplex ultrasound)
- Colour Doppler: Mean of velocities represented by colour scale
- Power Doppler: Amplitude of velocities, not direction, displayed
- Spectral Doppler: Range of velocities through time. Resistive index and pulsatility index used to calculate high and low resistance vessels

2) Artefacts

- Aliasing due to too low a PRF
- Spectral broadening due to turbulent flow and velocity being faster in centre of vessel
- Doppler angle must be <60° for accurate estimation
- Wall filter may remove genuine low velocities

4.6 US Artefacts

Image formation assumes:

- Sound travels in straight lines
- At a constant velocity
- With uniform attenuation
- Reflected only once from each interface

Artefacts result when the echo does not behave in this way and the system misinterprets it.

1) Acoustic Enhancement

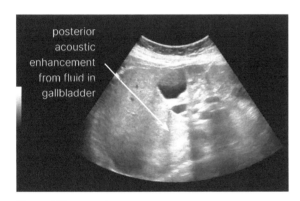

Figure 106 Acoustic enhancement

Fluid filled structures are weakly attenuating and a larger proportion and greater amplitude beam passes through to structures in the region behind. The machine interprets this as an increase in acoustic reflection and these structures show up brighter on the image.

2) Acoustic Shadowing

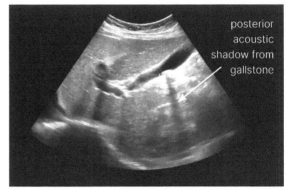

Figure 107 Acoustic shadowing

Hard calcific substances and soft tissue-air interfaces reflect almost all of the sound waves. No information is received from the area behind the structure.

3) Reverberation

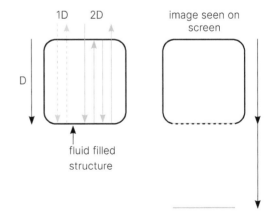

Figure 108 Reverberation artefact

Multiple reflections to and fro between the transducer face and a relatively strongly reflecting interface near the surface produces a series of delayed echoes. These look like stripes within a fluid filled structure.

Two types of reverberation artefact exist:
1. Comet tail: from metal or calcified objects
2. Ring down: from a collection of gas bubbles

4) Reflection / Mirror Artefact

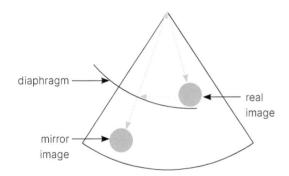

Figure 109 Mirror artefact

Sound bounces off a strongly reflecting object which acts as a mirror and reflects the pulse to another tissue interface. The interpretation of the image is that the second interface is beyond the first surface, much like the reverberation artefact. This most often happens at the diaphragm wherein the liver is seen in the chest cavity due to sound waves being reflected off the diaphragm.

5

Magnetic resonance imaging is one of the hardest subjects to understand in radiology physics, probably because most of the concepts are often oversimplified.

The first section of this chapter covers a little on the MR machine and the various magnets and coils as this will make it easier to understand the axes and how the transverse magnetisation is produced. This is then followed by an introduction to MRI which covers the basic physics of MR needed to understand everything else. We've subsequently separated out the physics of MR imaging in a way we found it easiest to work through and understand.

5.1   MR Machine   139

5.2   Introduction to MRI   141

5.3   T1 and T2 Signal   144

5.4   Spin Echo Sequence   148

5.5   T1, T2 and PD Weighted Imaging   151

5.6   Spatial Encoding   155

5.7   Slice Selection   157

5.8   Frequency Encoding   160

5.9   Phase Encoding   164

5.10 K-Space   166

5.11 Sequences   168

5.12 Spin Echo Sequences - Detailed   170

5.13 Gradient (Recalled) Echo Sequence   173

5.14 Inversion Recovery Sequences   175

5.15 Diffusion-Weighted Imaging   177

5.16 MR Spectroscopy   182

5.17 MR Angiography   185

5.18 MR Contrast Agents   190

5.19 MR Image Quality   192

5.20 MR Artefacts   196

5.21 MR Safety   202

5.1   MR Machine

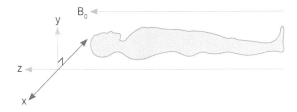

Figure 110 Axes of an MRI machine

A patient is placed in the bore of the MRI machine. The convention of the axes is shown above. These are the same axes as will be used throughout the MR notes.

There are several components to an MRI machine.

1) Superconducting electromagnet

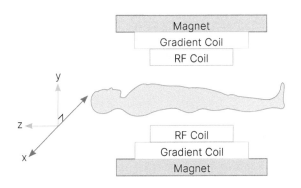

Figure 111 MRI machine magnets

A magnetic field, such as that created by a permanent magnet e.g. a bar magnet or fridge magnet you may have at home, is necessary for an MR machine to function. The problem is that for a bar magnet to create the field strength required, it would have to be massive. So, instead, we use a superconducting electromagnet. This is a magnet created by coils with an electric current running through it that then creates a magnetic field in the Z direction. This superconducting electromagnet is responsible for the main permanent magnetic field (B0) and weighs approx. 6 tonnes. It is always on.

The constant electric current generates a lot of heat and liquid helium (-269°C) is used to cool down the system. The helium also serves to reduce the resistance to the current being transmitted through the coils.

The majority of electromagnets create a magnetic field strength of 1.5 Tesla (T) or 3T. Some newer machines can generate fields of 7T. 1 Tesla = 10,000 gauss and the Earth's magnetic field is approx. 0.5 gauss (i.e. a 3 Tesla machine has a magnetic force of 60,000 times that of Earth).

2) Shim coils (not shown)

These lie just inside of the outer main magnet and are used to fine-tune the main magnetic field to ensure it is as uniform as possible.

3) Gradient coils

There are three sets of gradient coils orientated in the x, y and z axes used to alter the gradient of the magnetic field (the reason for this will become clear when reading about "Spatial Encoding"). The coils are switched on and off rapidly, in 1 ms or less, and it is this that creates the loud noise.

4) RF (radiofrequency) coils

These coils are tuned to a particular frequency. They produce a magnetic field at right angles (XY plane) to the main magnetic field and also receive the MR signals being produced. To maximise the signal the coils have to be placed as close to the part being imaged as possible. There are several types of RF coils:

1. Standard body coil (transmit and receive): permanent part of the scanner. Used to image large parts of the body
2. Head coil (transmit and receive): incorporated into a helmet and used for head scans
3. Surface (or local) coils (receive only): these are small coils applied as close to the area being imaged as possible e.g. arm, leg, orbits, lumbar spine coils etc.
4. Phased array coils: multiple receiver coils that receive the signals individually but are then combined to improve the signal-to-noise ratio
5. Transmit phased array coils

Now that we've covered the basics of the MR machine, we can go on to the introduction of MR physics.

5.2   Introduction to MRI

Hydrogen Nuclei as Magnets

A hydrogen nucleus contains a single proton so it has a charge of +1. The nucleus also has an intrinsic "spin". Because they have a charge and motion they create an electric current and this, in turn, creates a magnetic field. What this means is that hydrogen nuclei act like tiny magnets and will be affected by any magnetic field applied to them. Similarly, a magnetic field arising from tissue creates an electric current in the RF coils. In this way magnetic signals from tissue can be measured as an induced electric current in the RF coils of the MR machine.

Hydrogen nuclei are the most useful atoms to use in imaging mainly because they form the majority of atoms in the body. Any nucleus with an odd number of protons can be used (an unpaired proton is needed to provide the magnetic moment due to the spin of the un-paired proton).

Precession

As well as "spinning" about their own axis, when a magnetic field is applied the nuclei will "rotate" about the axis of the magnetic field. This is called **precession**. The example usually given is of a gyroscope or spinning

top. Spinning a gyroscope causes it to rotate about its own axis but gravity will also cause it to lean and spin about another axis dependent on the gravitational field strength.

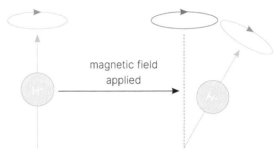

Figure 112 Precession

The frequency of this spinning is the **precessional / Larmor / rotational frequency**. In MR imaging we induce precession by applying a magnetic field (conventionally in the Z axis and called B_0, along the long axis of the patient). This magnetic field is permanently switched on in the MRI scanner.

The precessional frequency is calculated by the **Larmor Equation**

$$F = K \times B_0$$

Key: F = precessional frequency (Larmor frequency)

K = the gyromagnetic ratio (a constant that is different for different nuclei)

B_0 = strength of the static magnetic field

For a field strength of 1 Tesla the Larmor frequency of hydrogen is **42 Megahertz (MHz)** or 42 million cycles per second.

As the main magnetic field (B_0) is applied, the nuclei precess in the Z-axis along the applied magnetic field. Most will precess aligned with it (the low energy state) but a few will precess in the opposite direction (the high energy state). However, the majority will be aligned, creating a **net longitudinal magnetisation (Mz)** in the Z-axis direction.

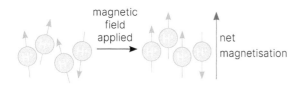

Figure 113 Net magnetisation in precession

Transverse Magnetisation

However, we cannot measure the longitudinal magnetisation and so we need to "**flip**" the magnetisation, usually to 90°, in order to be able to measure it and create our MRI signal. To flip the magnetisation a rapidly oscillating magnetic field at 90° to B_0 is applied (**B_1 / radiofrequency pulse / RF pulse**). This flips the net magnetisation into a **transverse plane (Mxy)**. In order to do this the B_1 magnetic field needs to oscillate at the same frequency as the precessing nuclei, the **resonant frequency**, as this ensures the most efficient trans-

ference of energy to the nuclei. Remember, this is 42 MHz for a 1 Tesla scanner and 63 MHz for a 1.5 Tesla scanner.

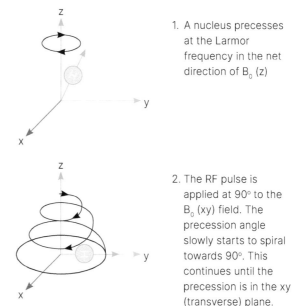

1. A nucleus precesses at the Larmor frequency in the net direction of B_0 (z)

2. The RF pulse is applied at 90° to the B_0 (xy) field. The precession angle slowly starts to spiral towards 90°. This continues until the precession is in the xy (transverse) plane.

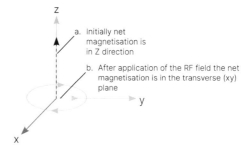

a. Initially net magnetisation is in Z direction

b. After application of the RF field the net magnetisation is in the transverse (xy) plane

3. As the nuclei spiral down, the magnetic direction of the nuclei line up and point in the same direction as they spin around (i.e. they are phase). This is what produces the net magnetisation and the "flip angle" of 90°.

Figure 114 Transverse magnetisation

Point of interest: why can't we measure longitudinal magnetisation?

1.   The net magnetisation vector is too small to measure when it is aligned with the

main magnetic field because the main field is so large.

2. When net magnetisation is at an angle to the main magnetic field, it precesses, and this generates a measureable signal perpendicular to the field.

Point of interest: radiofrequency pulse

For a 1.5T machine, the resonant frequency is 63 MHz which is within the range of radiowaves. Therefore, the exciting field (B_1) is called the radiofrequency or RF field.

Relaxation

As long as the RF pulse is applied the nuclei continue to precess in the transverse plane in phase creating a net transverse magnetisation (large Mxy). As soon as the RF is switched off, the transverse magnetisation begins to disappear and the nuclei relax back to their resting state of net longitudinal magnetisation (B_0, large Mz). This happens via two mechanisms and forms the basis for the T1 and T2 signals.

1. Spin-Lattice Relaxation or T_1 Recovery
2. Spin-Spin Relaxation or T_2 Decay

We will go into more detail in the next section.

5.3 T1 and T2 Signal

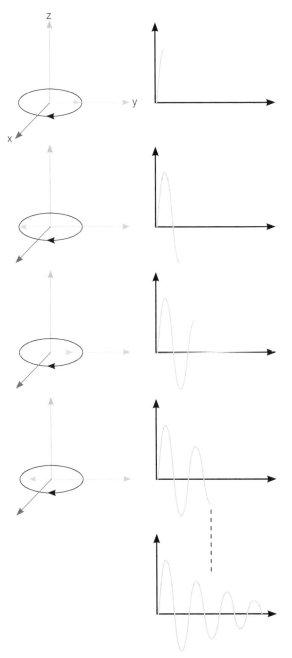

the nuclei in the xy plane in-phase, which creates a net magnetisation. This magnetisation precesses at the Larmor frequency inducing an electric voltage in the receiving coils. This electric signal is a sinusoidal wave of the same frequency as the net nuclei precession.

The signal is greatest during and immediately after the brief 90° RF pulse has been switched off. Then, the transverse magnetisation (Mxy) decays to zero and the longitudinal magnetisation (Mz) recovers to 100%. This consists of two different and independent mechanisms:

1. Spin-Lattice Relaxation
2. Spin-Spin Relaxation

Note:
It is important to note that these two processes are occurring at the same time but are completely independent i.e. the Mz of T1 recovers along a different time course to the Mxy of T2.

Figure 115 Transverse magnetisation and creation of signal

The MR signal is created by the precession of

Spin-Lattice Relaxation

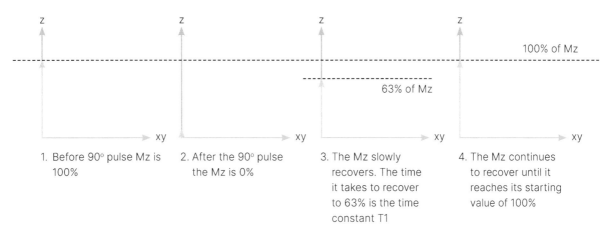

1. Before 90° pulse Mz is 100%
2. After the 90° pulse the Mz is 0%
3. The Mz slowly recovers. The time it takes to recover to 63% is the time constant T1
4. The Mz continues to recover until it reaches its starting value of 100%

Figure 116 T1 constant

As the nuclei precess in the transverse plane they are jostled by the surrounding molecules (i.e. the surrounding lattice) and they give up their energy to these molecules. As they do so they return to the longitudinal magnetisation (Mz) exponentially. This is called **Spin-Lattice** or **Longitudinal Relaxation**. The rate at which this happens is governed by the time constant **T1**.

- **T1** is the time it takes for Mz to recover to 63% of its maximum value.
- **T1** depends on the surrounding molecules and lattice.

*** T1 is always longer than T2 (except water in which T1 = T2) ***

Note: The 90° RF pulse will pull all the Mz signal to 90° i.e. to the Mxy plane. This means if we have a large Mz signal then apply a 90° RF pulse, it becomes an Mxy signal of the same magnitude. We will ignore this for the moment as we are only focusing on the Mz signal which is zero, but we will come back to it when we look at weighted imaging.

Effects on T1

Fat and protein: short T1. The molecules are large with low innate energy. This makes them very effective at absorbing energy causing a quick loss of Mxy and, therefore, quick recovery of Mz and a short T1.

Water: long T1. The molecules are small and move quickly making them inefficient at jostling the nuclei and absorbing energy. This causes a long T1.

Bone / calcium / metal: very long T1. The macromolecules are fixed and rigid and are the least effective at removing energy from the precessing nuclei.

*** Fast food (fat causes short T1) and long drink of water (water causes long T1) ***

Spin-Spin Relaxation

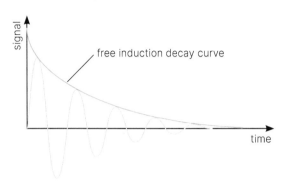

Figure 117 Free induction decay curve

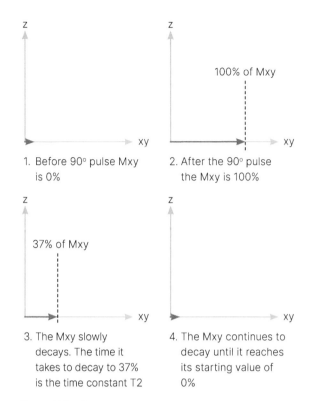

1. Before 90° pulse Mxy is 0%

2. After the 90° pulse the Mxy is 100%

100% of Mxy

37% of Mxy

3. The Mxy slowly decays. The time it takes to decay to 37% is the time constant T2

4. The Mxy continues to decay until it reaches its starting value of 0%

Figure 118 T2 constant

Once the RF pulse is stopped, the magnetic properties of each nuclei alter the local magnetic field and cause some to precess faster and some slower (remember, the precessional, or Larmor frequency, is determined by the strength of the magnetic field).

Gradually the nuclei lose their coherence and the net transverse magnetisation reduces to zero. The rate it does so is exponential and called the "**Free Induction Decay**".

The rate at which the transverse magnetisation is lost is determined by the magnetic interaction between the spins and is called the **spin-spin** or **transverse decay**. The time constant of this fall-off is called the **T2**.

- **T2** is the time it takes for the transverse magnetisation to decay to 37% of its value (i.e. loses 63% of its maximum signal)
- **T2** depends on the local magnetic field.

Effects on T2

Bone / calcium / metal: short T2. The local variation of magnetic field is greatest in solids and macromolecules that are rigid.

Fat: Short T2.

Water: Very long T2. The lighter molecules are in rapid thermal motion that smoothes out the local field producing a longer T2.

1) T2* or free induction decay

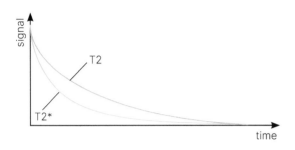

Figure 119 T2 star signal

	T1 (ms)	T2 (ms)
Fat	250	80
Kidney	550	60
White matter	650	90
Grey matter	800	100
CSF	2000	150
Water	3000	3000
Bone, teeth	Very long	Very short

What has just been described is the exponential curve of transverse decay in the ideal world. However, when we measure it in the real world we find that the transverse decay is much quicker; the signal reduces to zero faster than expected. This is called the T2* curve.

This is due to the effect of the local and external magnetic field inhomogeneities. Although the B_0 magnetic field is largely the same throughout it is not exactly homogeneous and the tissue and other materials within the magnetic field will also affect the magnetic field. This variation causes the nuclei to dephase quicker.

The **spin-echo sequence** explained next deletes the effect of local field inhomogeneities so that only the tissue characteristic T2 effect is recorded.

T1 and T2 Values

Relaxation times of different tissues in a magnetic field of 1 Tesla:

Summary

- T1 recovery
  - Due to spin-lattice relaxation
  - Recovery of longitudinal magnetisation (Mz)
  - T1 time constant is time it takes to recover 63% of maximum Mz
- T2 decay
  - Due to spin-spin decay
  - Decay of transverse magnetisation (Mxy)
  - T2 time constant is time it takes to decay to 37% of maximum Mxy
- T2* / Free Induction Decay
  - T2 decay due to superimposed magnetic field inhomogeneities
  - T2* shorter than T2
- T1 vs T2
  - Water: long T1, very long T2
  - Fat: short T1, short T2
  - T1 is always longer than T2 except in pure water in which T1=T2

5.4   Spin Echo Sequence

There are many sequences used in MRI, each one aimed at increasing the tissue contrast of interest. The basic sequences are:

1. Spin echo
2. Gradient echo

We will first go through the spin echo sequence. A spin echo sequence aims to remove the effects of the static field (T2*) but leave the tissue characteristic T2 effect.

Application of 90° RF Pulse

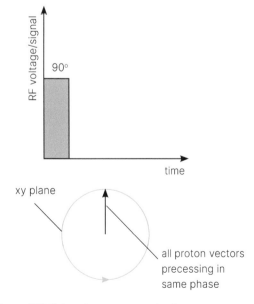

Figure 120 Spin echo sequence step 1

3. A 90° RF pulse is applied. All proton vectors precess in phase and the Mxy signal is at its maximum.

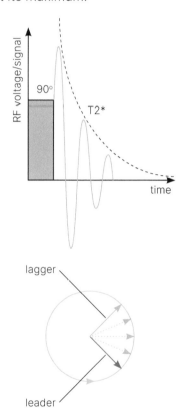

Figure 121 Spin echo sequence step 2

4. The Mxy signal decays rapidly due to the T2* or free induction decay. There are some proton vectors that are fast and lead and some that are slow and lag as they dephase.

Application of 180° RF Rephasing Pulse

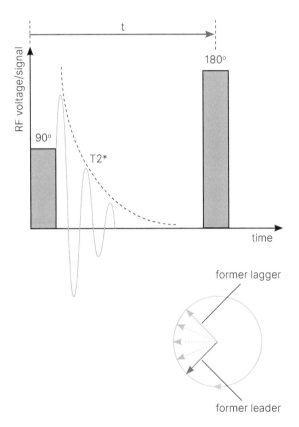

Figure 122 Spin echo sequence step 3

1. After a time (t) a 180° RF pulse is applied. This is simply a pulse that is applied twice as long as the 90° pulse in the transverse plane. All proton vectors are turned through 180°. The laggers become leaders and vice-versa.

Echo

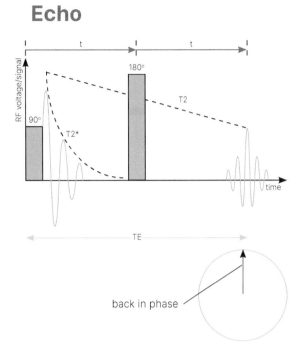

Figure 123 Spin echo sequence step 4

2. After the same amount of time (t) the proton vectors are again in phase, the Mxy signal is at its peak. This is the **echo** and this is the signal that is measured. The decay in the signal from the original 90° to the echo is due to the tissue characteristic T2 effect with the effect of magnetic field inhomogeneities minimised.

The time at which this echo is produced is the **TE** (time to echo). It is produced at exactly 2t, t being the time at which the 180° RF pulse is applied (i.e. the 180° RF pulse is applied at **TE/2**). The mechanism through which the echo is created is gone into in more detail in the diagram below.

1. The 90° RF pulse causes all protons to precess in phase.

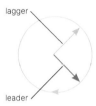

2. After the 90° RF pulse is removed, the protons start to dephase - some quickly and some slowly. For simplicity only two proton vectors are shown.

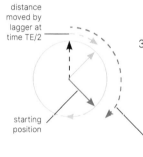

3. At time TE/2, the 180° RF pulse is applied. At this point the laggers and leaders have moved out of phase by a certain amount.

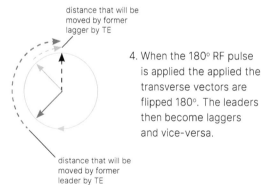

4. When the 180° RF pulse is applied the applied the transverse vectors are flipped 180°. The leaders then become laggers and vice-versa.

5. At TE the vectors will return to be in phase. The Mxy will be maximum and the echo will be produced.

Figure 124 Spin echo sequence in detail

Repeat Cycle

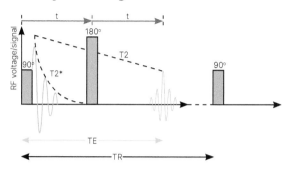

Figure 125 Spin echo sequence step 5

5. One cycle has now been completed. This cycle is repeated hundreds of times in the sequence. The time to the next cycle is **TR** (time to repetition).

Summary

1. Initial 90° RF pulse
2. At TE/2, 180° pulse applied
3. At TE, echo signal measured
4. Cycle repeated after TR

Advantages	Disadvantage
High SNR True T2 weighting Minimise susceptibility effects	Long scan times Uses more RF power than a GE

There is more to a spin echo than we covered above, and we will go into more detail in 5.12 - Spin Echo Sequences - Detailed. For the moment, however, lets go through how to create weighted images by altering the parameters of sequences.

5.5　T1, T2 and PD Weighted Imaging

Unlike imaging using radiation, in which the contrast depends on the different attenuation of the structures being imaged, the contrast in MR images depends on the magnetic properties and number of hydrogen nuclei in the area being imaged. Different contrasts in the area being imaged can be selected for by running different sequences with different weightings. The main three sequences are:

1. T1-weighted (maximum T1 contrast shown)
2. T2-weighted (maximum T2 contrast shown)
3. Proton density (PD) weighting (density of hydrogen protons shown)

There are other more complicated sequences as well (e.g. fluid attenuated inversion recovery (FLAIR) and short tau inversion recovery (STIR)) which we will cover later.

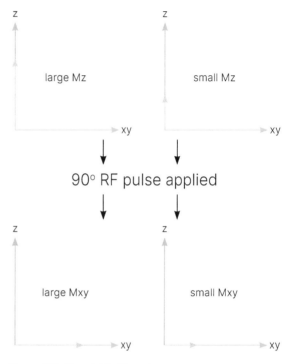

Figure 126 T1 weighted imaging

T1-Weighted Imaging

To recap, T1 relaxation is the recovery of the longitudinal magnetisation (Mz). The higher the Mz at the time of applying the 90° RF pulse the greater the transverse signal (Mxy).

The TR (time to repetition) is what determines the length of time between 90° RF pulses:

The longer the TR
↓
The longer the time to the next 90° RF pulse
↓
The more time Mz will have had to recover
↓
The higher the transverse signal when the 90° RF pulse is applied

*** i.e. it is the TR that determines the T1 signal ***

The time constant, T1, is a measure of the time it takes for the nuclei to reach 63% of their original Mz. Hydrogen nuclei in different molecules have different T1s. Those with a short T1 will recover their Mz quicker than those with a long T1.

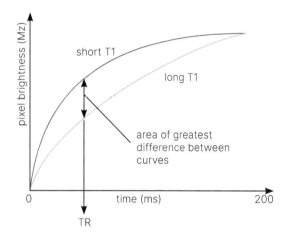

Figure 127 T1 weighted imaging

To maximise the contrast between the T1 properties of tissues in the sample being imaged, we need to set the TR so that it occurs at the point in the curve at which there is the greatest difference. As seen on the curve above, this is at a **short TR**.

1) Note about T2 weighted imaging

In order to maximise T2 weighted imaging we want to minimise the contribution of T1 contrast. Looking at the above chart, the smallest T1 contrast is at long or short TR's. At short TR's the signal is too small to be of use and so a **long TR** is used.

T2-Weighted Imaging

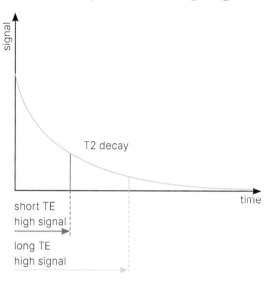

Figure 128 T2 weighted imaging

To recap, T2 decay is the decay of the transverse magnetisation (Mxy) after application of the 90° RF pulse.

The longer the time after the 90° RF pulse, the more the Mxy decays and the smaller the transverse signal. As we saw in the spin echo sequence, TE is the "time to echo". If we have a long TE there is more time for the Mxy to decay and we get a smaller signal.

The longer the TE
↓
The longer the time allowed for Mxy to decay
↓
The smaller the transverse (T2) signal

*** i.e. it is the TE that determines the T2 signal ***

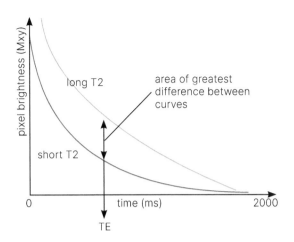

Figure 129 T2 weighted imaging

The time constant, T2, is the time it takes for the signal to decay to 37% of its excited Mxy. Hydrogen nuclei in different molecules have different T2's. Those with a short T2 will take a shorter time to decay than those with a long T2.

To maximise the T2 contrast a **long TE** is used, although not so long that the signal is negligible.

2) Note About T1 Weighted Imaging

To maximise the T1 signal in T1-weighted imaging we want to minimise the contribution of the T2 signal. From figure 128 we see that the smallest contrast occurs at a small TE or a very long TE. However, at very long TE's the signal is too small and so a **short TE** is used in T1 weighted imaging.

Proton Density Imaging

Unlike T1 and T2 weighted images, proton density (PD) does not display the magnetic characteristics of the hydrogen nuclei but the **number** of nuclei in the area being imaged. To get a PD weighted image we want to minimise the contribution of both T1 and T2 contrast.

- T1 minimised with a long TR: large signal and small T1 contrast
- T2 minimised with a short TE: large signal and small T2 contrast

Summary

	T1	T2	PD
Image			
Water signal	Water has a long T1. T1-WI uses a short TR so the signal from water is still low, therefore, water appears **dark**	T2-WI uses a long TE so the signal from water is high, therefore, water appears **bright**	A long TR results in a high water signal, but a short TE means that this is less than the signal of a T2 scan. The signal of water is in the middle
Fat signal	Fat has a short T1, so even though the TR is short the signal is still high and fat appears **bright**	Fat has a short T2, so at a long TE the signal is **less bright** and it will be darker than water, but still high	A long TR results in a high fat signal and short TE means this signal is higher than on a T2-WI. Fat appears **bright**
TR	Short. 300-600 ms	Long. 2000 ms	Long. 1000-3000 ms
TE	Short. 10-30 ms	Long. 90-140 ms	Short. 15 ms

5.6   Spatial Encoding

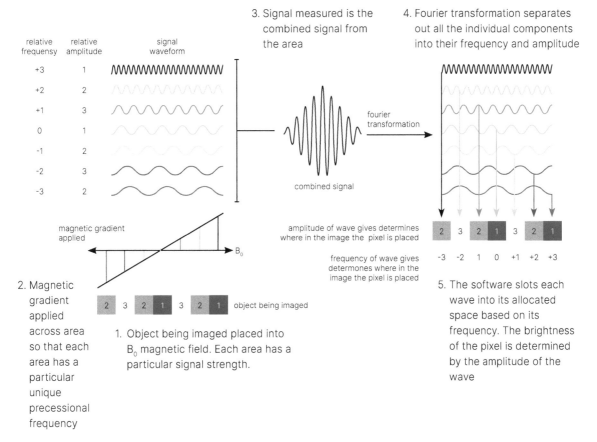

3. Signal measured is the combined signal from the area

4. Fourier transformation separates out all the individual components into their frequency and amplitude

relative frequensy | relative amplitude | signal waveform

+3 | 1
+2 | 2
+1 | 3
0 | 1
-1 | 2
-2 | 3
-3 | 2

fourier transformation

combined signal

magnetic gradient applied

B_0

amplitude of wave gives determines where in the image the pixel is placed

frequency of wave gives determones where in the image the pixel is placed

2 | 3 | 2 | 1 | 3 | 2 | 1

-3 -2 1 0 +1 +2 +3

2. Magnetic gradient applied across area so that each area has a particular unique precessional frequency

2 | 3 | 2 | 1 | 3 | 2 | 1   object being imaged

1. Object being imaged placed into B_0 magnetic field. Each area has a particular signal strength.

5. The software slots each wave into its allocated space based on its frequency. The brightness of the pixel is determined by the amplitude of the wave

Figure 130 Spatial encoding

Unlike in CT and plain films in which localisation of the signal is simple (an x-ray beam travels through the material and where it hits the receptor is the physical location of what it has passed through) MRI is much more complicated. With MRI the signal is localised in the 3D space by manipulating the magnetic properties of the nuclei in a predictable way. The signals are then returned with a particular frequency and phase and these are slotted into their respective locations.

The brightness of the pixel is the amplitude of the signal returned. The key concept of spatial encoding is the use of gradients.

There are three steps involved in identifying where in a 3D location a signal is arising from:
1. Slice selected along z-axis
2. Segment of slice along x-axis selected by **frequency encoding**
3. Part of segment along y-axis selected by **phase encoding**

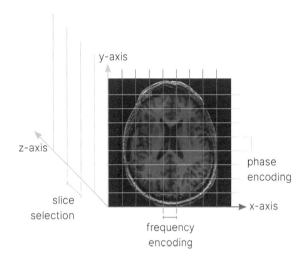

y-axis

z-axis

slice
selection

phase
encoding

x-axis

frequency
encoding

Figure 131 Spatial localisation

5.7 Slice Selection

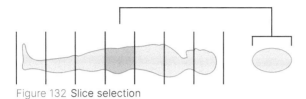

Figure 132 Slice selection

The first part of localising the signal is to localise it the location of the axial slice within the object being imaged. This is known as "**slice selection**". The way this is done is by using the RF pulse to select which slice to activate i.e. which slice will have the magnetic vector of its nuclei flipped to the transverse plane in order to return a signal.

A magnetic field gradient is applied in the Z-axis superimposed on the background magnetic field. Going back to the Larmor equation the frequency of precession depends on the magnetic field. This means that nuclei will have different frequencies throughout the z-axis.

2) Select slice

An RF pulse is applied to flip the magnetisation of the nuclei into the transverse plane and, therefore, give a signal. Remember, to flip the precession of the nuclei the RF pulse frequency should be the same as the Larmor frequency of the nuclei. As the Larmor frequency of nuclei is different along the z-axis we can select a slice to activate by altering the frequency of the RF pulse.

Slice Selection

1) Apply gradient

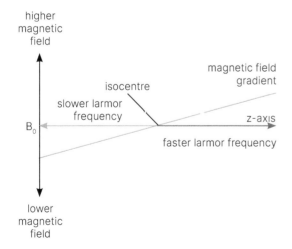

Figure 133 Selecting slice with gradient

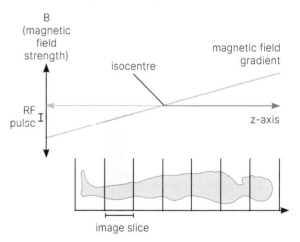

Figure 134 Selecting slice 1

3) Reset

As the frequencies are different along the gradient, the nuclei begin to precess out of phase. Before selecting the next slice we need to reset the nuclei. This is done by temporarily reversing the gradient to reverse the precessional frequencies. The nuclei then re-phase.

1. No gradient applied. All nuclei precessing at same frequency and phase.

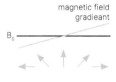

2. Gradient applied, the Larmar frequency of the nuclei is along a gradient. As the frequencies are different they get out of phase.

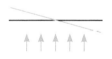

3. The gradient is reserved. Those that had the highest frequency now have the lowest and vice versa. The phases catch up until they are reset.

Figure 135 Resetting the gradient

4) Summary

1. A magnetic field gradient is applied in the z-axis
2. The Larmor frequencies of the nuclei vary along the z-axis
3. An RF pulse with a frequency matching the Larmor frequency of the nuclei we want to select is applied
4. In this way, a slice along the z-axis is selected (correlates with an axial slice of the patient)
5. The phases of the nuclei are reset by reversing the gradients

Factors Affecting Slice Properties

1) RF pulse bandwidth

The RF pulse bandwidth is the range of frequencies within the pulse

Large bandwidth = large range of frequencies = larger slice

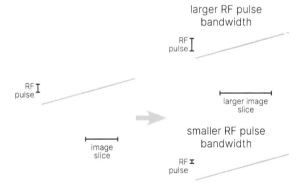

Figure 136 Slice selection - Changing RF bandwidth

2) RF pulse frequency

Changing the RF pulse frequency moves the slice selected up and down the z-axis.

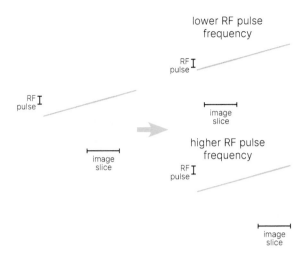

Larger gradient = smaller image slice

Smaller gradient = larger image slice

Figure 137 Slice selection - changing pulse frequency

3) Gradient strength

Altering the gradient strength alters the steepness of the gradient. The same RF pulse will then activate (select) a different size of slice

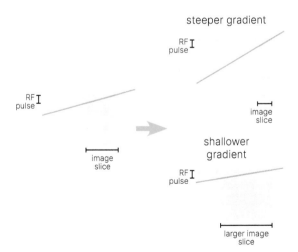

Figure 138 Slice selection - gradient strength

5.8 Frequency Encoding

Read-Out Gradient

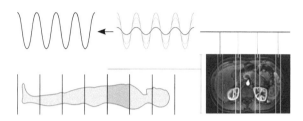

Figure 130 Readout gradient 1

We have now selected a slice by applying a gradient in the z-axis. Should we want to select a section of the slice in the x-axis (i.e. a column), all nuclei along the x-axis of the slice will have different amplitudes (indicating different brightness values) but they will have the same frequency and phase. Adding all the signals together results in one large wave of the same frequency. This is of no use if we want to localise the signal in the x-axis as all locations will have the same frequency.

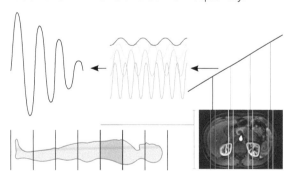

Figure 140 Readout gradient 2

We overcome this by applying another magnetic gradient in the x-axis. This changes the Larmor frequencies of the nuclei in a gradient along the x-axis. Each segment will now return a signal of a different frequency depending on its location along the slice. As they are of different frequencies, they will eventually become of different phases. Adding the signals together gives a large signal at the start, when they are still all in phase, but this signal drops off as the phases diverge.

This gradient is called the "**read out**" or "**frequency encoding**" gradient.

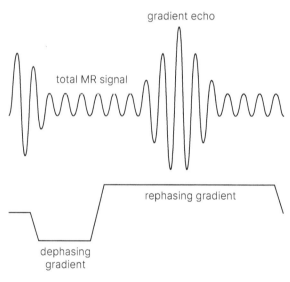

Figure 141 Rephasing the signal

One of the consequences of the gradient is that as the signals go out of phase the total signal becomes very small leaving a small amount of time in which a useful signal can be measured. To overcome this, a "**dephase**" gradient is first applied.

The read-out gradient then rephases the MR signals such that they all come back into phase and form the maximum signal during the data collection period - the **gradient echo**.

Usually, the dephasing and read-out gradients are designed so that the gradient echo occurs in the middle of the data collection period.

1) Decoding the signal

Now we have one MR signal formed of many MR signals of different frequencies. Luckily, we can easily extract out each frequency and its amplitude mathematically using the **Fourier Transformation (FT)**.

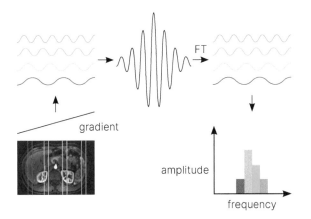

Figure 142 Decoding the signal

We can now map each signal to its location in the x-axis of the slice by its frequency and assign the corresponding amplitude (brightness).

Artefacts from Frequency Encoding

1) Aliasing

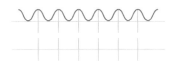

if the sampling frequency is 1 Hz (one sample per second), for a wave of 1 Hz (1 wave per second) the frequency is accurately recorded as 1 Hz

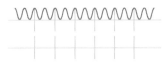

for a wave of 2 Hz the frequency is underestimated to be 1 Hz as the sampling frequency is not high enough

Figure 143 Aliasing in frequency encoding

The wave signal we receive has to be digitised before the FT can be applied and the frequencies extracted via **sampling**. If the signal is not sampled regularly enough, we will underestimate its frequency - this is called **aliasing**. The sampling frequency required to give an accurate result can be calculated with the **Nyquist limit** i.e. the maximum signal frequency that can be accurately sampled:

Nyquist limit = sampling frequency / 2

A high frequency signal is wrongly sampled as a low frequency signal and slotted into the low frequency location resulting in wrap-around.

To ensure that this limit is not surpassed the range of frequencies is limited prior to sampling using a **'band-pass filter'** that will only allow through a certain range of frequencies - the **receiver bandwidth**. The edges of the field-of-view in the frequency-encoding direction correspond to limits of the receiver bandwidth.

Overcoming aliasing
- Larger field of view (FOV)
- Use pre-saturation bands on the areas outside the FOV to null the signal
- Anti-aliasing software
- Switch phase and frequency directions
- Use surface coil - these are sensitive only to the areas in the FOV and also improve signal-to-noise ratio

2) Chemical shift

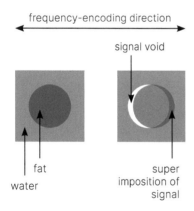

frequency-encoding direction

signal void

fat

water

super imposition of signal

Figure 144 Chemical shift artefact

In frequency-encoding we assume that all nuclei will have the same Larmor frequency. However, nuclei in fat and water will have slightly different frequencies due to the local magnetic field effects. This difference in frequencies due to different environments is **misregistered** as differences due to location.

This artefact only occurs in the frequency-encoding direction.

Factors affecting chemical shift
- Chemical shift increases with magnetic field strength
    - relatively greater difference between the frequencies
- Chemical shift increases with decreasing gradient strength
    - shallower gradient means more frequencies coded within the same area, small differences in frequencies will be more evident
- Narrower bandwidth gives higher chemical shift
    - same reasoning as above

Summary

1. Gradient applied in z-axis to select axial slice
2. Dephase gradient applied along x-axis
3. Rephase read-out gradient applied along x-axis
4. Gradient echo signal received (combination of all signals along the x-axis)
5. Fourier transfer applied to combined signals
6. Signals separated out by frequency:
    - Each frequency relates to location along x-axis

- Each frequency's amplitude gives the signal brightness

5.9   Phase Encoding

Now that we have selected a single slice and a single column within that slice, we need to localise the signal along that column (ie. the row). We do this by applying another gradient in the y-axis.

1) Apply phase-encoding gradient

If we take a single column through the slice (i.e. a single frequency in the read-out direction) and then divide this into sections in the y-axis, each segment will have the same frequency and phase.

We switch on the phase-encoding gradient along the y-axis before the readout gradient. Some sections will precess with a quicker frequency and some with a slower frequency. When we switch off the gradient all the segments return to the same frequency but they are now all out of phase with a phase-shift that depends on the position along the column.

2) Repeat cycle

With every cycle the amplitude of the phase encoding gradient is changed so that the phase of the MR signal at a certain y-axis position changes each time. If we look at a single point in time along the cycle and look at the amplitude of the wave at that point, it varies with each cycle. If we then plot this amplitude with each cycle we get another wave.

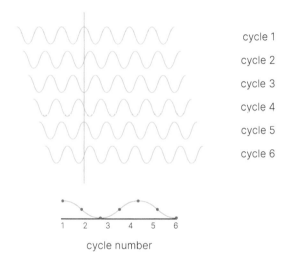

Figure 145 Phase encoding repeat cycle

Each point along the segment will have a phase encoding curve with a different frequency. Those at the furthest ends of the gradient will have a greater change in their phases and, therefore, a higher frequency phase encoding curve. The point at the middle of the gradient, the isopoint, will never change its frequency or, therefore, its phase. A Fourier transform is again applied to extract these frequencies and place them in the correct place along the y-axis.

The signal strength (brightness) is given by the maximum amplitude of the phase-shift curve as this corresponds to the maximum amplitude of the original signal.

Summary

1. Phase-encoding gradient applied along y-axis
2. The frequencies of each segment in the column are now different
3. Gradient switched off
4. The frequencies return to the frequency of that column (as determined by the frequency-encoding gradient)
5. However, they are now out of phase
6. The amplitude of the signals is plotted
7. The cycle is repeated with different strengths of phase-encoding gradients producing different phase shifts each time
8. The plot of the amplitude with each phase shift forms a wave with a particular frequency
9. Each area in the column with have a phase-shift wave with a different frequency depending upon its area along the y-axis
10. Fourier transform is applied to separate out the frequencies and slot them into their position along the y-axis

5.10 K-Space

As we acquire our images, what we are acquiring is many, many waves of varying spatial frequency and directions. As we overlay these on top of one another we form the physical image. These wave signals are stored in K-Space (aka Fourier Space) along a coordinate system.

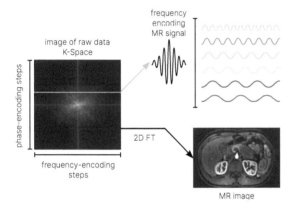

Figure 146 K-space

Each column of k-space contains the data obtained during one frequency encoding step. Each row is filled in by repeating the phase-encoding steps. The important things to note are:

- Any particular point on K-space contributes to the whole image
- Any image pixel is derived from the whole of K-space
- K-space is symmetrical

Within K-space the high-frequency signals are within the periphery and the low-frequency signals are within the centre. The x and y-axes determine the orientation of the signal wavelengths.

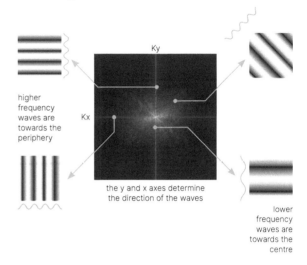

Figure 147 Example of wave signals in K-space

A low-pass filter that only includes the centre of K-space produces an image that is very smooth but lacks the edges and details. A high-pass filter that only includes the periphery of K-space produces an image that has very good detail and edges but no low-contrast features.

Original input and the K-space map

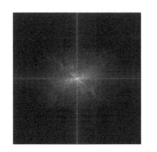 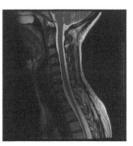

Figure 148 Input image of K-space

High-pass filter

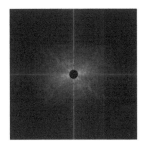 

Figure 149 High-pass filter

Low-pass filter

 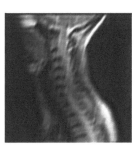

Figure 150 Low-pass filter

- High-frequency signals (edges) are stored in the periphery
- Low-frequency signals (contrast) are stored in the centre

Summary

- The wavelength signals acquired are stored in K-space
- Each column contains data acquired from 1 frequency encoding step
- Each row contains data acquired from phase-encoding steps
- Any point in K-space contributes to the whole image
- Any image pixel is derived from the whole of K-space

5.11 Sequences

Now that we know about more of the components of a sequence (slice selection etc), we can look further into the anatomy of a sequence.

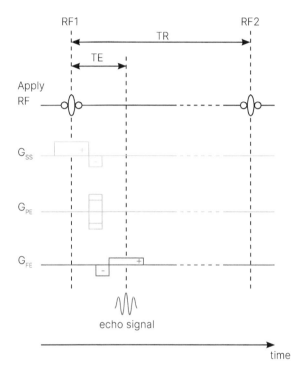

Figure 151 Anatomy of an MRI sequence

1) Step 1 - RF Pulse

An RF pulse is applied to flip the magnetisation into the transverse plane. The RF pulse is usually represented as a 'sinc' shape to indicate the envelope of the RF pulse.

2) Step 2 - Slice Selection (G_{SS})

The RF pulse must be applied at the same time as a slice-select gradient in order to excite the protons in a particular slice.

The area of the negative lobe of the gradient is equal to half the area of the positive lobe to ensure phase coherence is maintained within the image slice.

3) Step 3 - Phase Encoding (G_{PE})

This is applied straight after the RF excitation and slice selection has been completed. The cycle has to be repeated the same number of times as rows in the k-space. Each time, a different phase-encoding gradient is used and a different line is filled. The steps of the phase encoding gradient symbol represent the different strengths of the gradient applied. For simplicity, we have only shown 5 steps although there are typically 256 or 512 depending on the matrix size.

4) Step 4 - Frequency Encoding (G_{FE})

The frequency-encoding gradient is applied after each step of the phase encoding gradient and it is during the gradient that the signal is 'read' (hence the alternative name of 'readout gradient'). From the notes on FE gradient an opposite dephasing gradient is applied first then the rephasing gradient in order to create an echo with a large enough signal.

The negative dephasing gradient is half the area of the rephasing gradient in order to ensure the phase coherence is maximal at the central point of the frequency encoding and, therefore, the acquired signal will be maximal.

5) Step 5 - Sequence Repetition

After a time (TR) the whole sequence is repeated again with a new RF pulse. The number of times this is repeated depends on the image resolution and the number of phase-encoding steps required.

Key point

The number of phase-encoding steps determines the number of lines in k-space and, hence, the resolution (e.g. 512 phase encoding steps gives a resolution of 512 in the y-axis)

The scan time = TR x number of phase-encoding steps x NEX

(NEX = number of signal averages)

We can now go into more detail on different sequences.

5.12 Spin Echo Sequences - Detailed

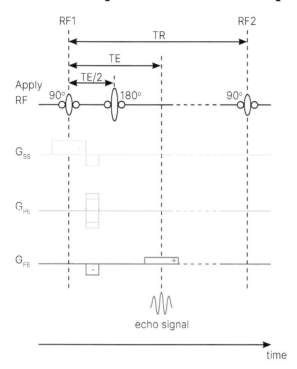

Figure 152 Spin echo sequence

prior to the 180° RF pulse. This has the same effect as a negative FE gradient applied after the 180° pulse.

Multi-Slice Sequence

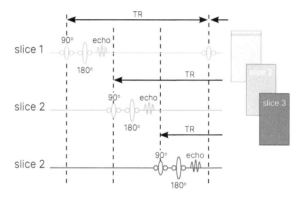

Figure 153 Multislice sequence

We have already covered the spin echo sequence in some detail earlier. The difference between this sequence and the one outlined on the previous page is the addition of the 180° RF pulse at TE/2.

In the previous sequence and in gradient echo sequences the signal decays quickly due to magnetic field inhomogeneities. The spin echo sequence preserves the MRI signal for longer with the addition of the 180° pulse as described previously.

The second difference is the frequency-encoding gradient. A positive gradient is applied

The length of the TR needs to allow sufficient time for the T1 relaxation to complete in order to have enough Mz to give a signal when it is flipped by the 90° pulse.

If a scan contains 18 slices:
- The TR is 540ms
- A matrix size of 256 × 512 (256 phase encoding steps are required per slice)
- The scan time is:

TR x PE steps x Number of slices / 60,000

540 × 256 × 18 / 60,000 = 41.4 minutes

Considering the TE is only 30ms, this is a very long scan with a lot of dead time in which no signal is being created. We can use this dead time by selecting another slice and starting a cycle, then selecting a third slice and starting a cycle etc. After 540 ms it is time to start the second cycle for the first slice. In 540 ms we can scan 18 lines of 18 different k-spaces. Now we just need to repeat this enough times to get every line of every k-space (i.e. multiply by the number of phase-encoding steps). Recalculating the scan time gives us:

$$540 \times 256 / 60{,}000 = 2.3 \text{ minutes}$$

This technique is used in nearly every scan to make the scan times shorter.

Multi Echo Sequence

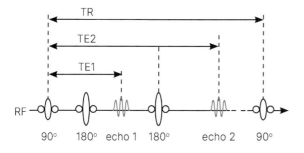

Figure 154 Multiecho sequence

So far, only one echo per cycle is being created. We can acquire more echoes in one cycle.

From chapter 5.5 - T1, T2 and PD Weighted Imaging we saw that by selecting different TEs we can create different weighted images:

- PD weighted uses a short TE of 15 ms
- T2 weighted uses a long TE of 1000-3000 ms

We can transmit two 180° pulses to create two echoes with different TEs of the same row of the same k-space. In this way, we create a PD and a T2 image in the same amount of time as it takes to create one image.

Turbo Spin Echo (TSE) Sequence

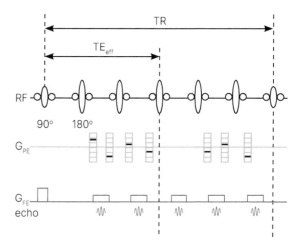

Figure 155 Turbo spin echo sequence

We can take the multi-echo sequence further. We can repeat the 180° RF pulses many times, creating many echoes, within one cycle. If we apply a different G_{PE} each time we can fill up different lines of k-space. The number of echoes we create is called the "**echo train length (ETL)**". In the above example, the ETL is 5 but we can use an ETL of 212. The TE measured is taken to be the echo created when the G_{PE}

is zero and is called the "**effective TE (T$_{eff}$)**".

N.B. The phase-encoding gradient is reversed prior to the next 180° RF pulse to rephase the spins.

This will shorten the sequence time:

Normal spin echo = TR x no. G$_{PE}$ x number of slices

Turbo spin echo = TR x no. G$_{PE}$ x number of slices / ETL

Advantages

- Very fast - useful for MR angiography in which very fast scan times are needed.
- Can create two images of different contrasts by filling two different k-spaces, e.g. if we have an ETL of 14, we can use the first 7 echoes for a PD image (first k-space) and the last 7 echoes for a T2 image (second k-space). This is called a Double-Echo TSE sequence

Disadvantages

- Only really able to achieve heavily T2 weighted images
- Mix of contrasts: Each echo that fills a different line of k-space is at a different time and, therefore, a different contrast.

Echo or HASTE Sequence

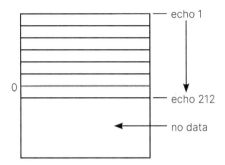

Figure 156 Haste sequence

We can take the TSE one step further and fill an entire k-space in one cycle. If we use an ETL of 212 it reduces the scan times significantly. Furthermore, we only really need to fill up just over half of k-space (i.e. 212 rows). We can then use a Half Fourier Imaging to extrapolate the rest of k space and complete the image.

The very late echoes are put in the centre of k-space (heavily T2 weighted) which results in an image that only shows free water. This is the sequence used in an MRCP study.

We've now gone through one type of sequence - the Spin Echo sequence. Next, we'll cover Gradient Echo sequences.

Fast Advanced Spin

5.13 Gradient (Recalled) Echo Sequence

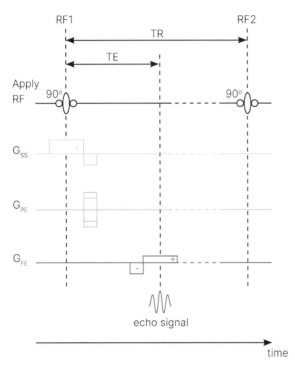

Figure 157 Gradient echo sequence

Spin echo sequences work fine for sequences of a long TR. If a short TR is needed (for example, in T1 weighted scans), we need to cut down the scan time. We do this by forgoing the 180° RF pulse and, instead, using a gradient to rephase the spins. This is a gradient echo sequence.

1. RF pulse applied
2. Slice-select gradient applied
3. Phase-encoding gradient applied
4. Frequency-encoding gradient applied
   - A negative G_{FE} is applied. The spins dephase, some faster than others.
   - The positive G_{FE} is applied. The spins start to rephase until they are again in phase and a signal is created - the **Gradient Echo**

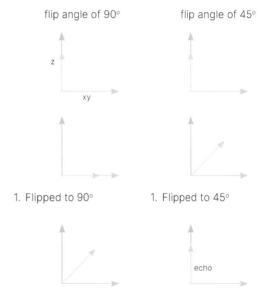

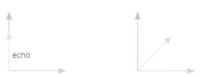

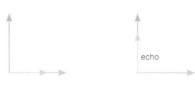

flip angle of 90°	flip angle of 45°
1. Flipped to 90°	1. Flipped to 45°
2. After time (t), the 90° flip angle has only recovered half-way	2. After time (t), the 45° flip angle has returned to maximum Mz and we can reflip it.
2. After time (2t), the 90° flip angle has now fully recovered its Mz and we can re-flip it now	3. Flipped to 45°
4. Flipped to 90°	
one echo generated	**two echos generated**

Figure 158 Flip angle in gradient echo

The other aspect of a GRE sequence is that you don't have to use a 90° RF pulse at the start of the cycle, an RF pulse of any flip angle can be used. If an RF pulse with a smaller flip angle is used, it will take less time for the spins to regain all their Mz as they are closer to 0°. However, this also means that the Mxy signal is not as high as if a 90° flip angle was used.

	PD	T1w	T2*w	T2
Flip angle	Small angle	Large angle	Small angle (minimise T1w)	Can't achieve T2w as no 180° RF pulses to cancel T2* effect
TE	Short	Short	Long	
TR	Long	Short	Short	

Weighting Using GRE Sequences

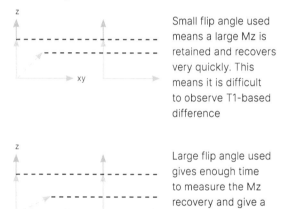

Small flip angle used means a large Mz is retained and recovers very quickly. This means it is difficult to observe T1-based difference

Large flip angle used gives enough time to measure the Mz recovery and give a T1-weighted image

Figure 159 Lage and small flip angle

Summary

Spin echo	Gradient echo
RF pulse used to rephase	Gradient applied to rephase
Uses flip angle of 90°	Uses variable flip angle
Slow sequence	Fast sequence
True T2 weighting	T2* weighting - susceptible to magnetic field inhomogeneities

5.14 Inversion Recovery Sequences

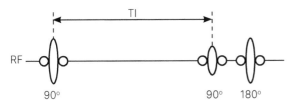

Figure 160 Inversion recovery sequence

Inversion recovery sequences are a variant of Spin Echo sequences. They are used to null the signal from certain tissues, e.g. fat in a STIR and fluid in a FLAIR, by first applying a 180° RF pulse and then starting the cycle.

This flips the Mz through 180° to a negative value. As the Mz recovers, at some point it reaches zero before becoming positive again. If we apply our 90° RF pulse when the Mz is 0, at time **TI (time to inversion)**, there is no magnetisation to create a Mxy signal. We have, in effect, nulled that signal. The TI (time from initial inverting 180° pulse to the subsequent 90° pulse) is altered based upon the material that we want to null the signal from.

As fat and fluid have different T1s and will reach Mz of zero at different times, we can select which tissue to null by selecting when to start the 90° RF pulse.

1) STIR (Short Tau Inversion Recovery)

Fat signal nulled by selecting short TI (130 ms)

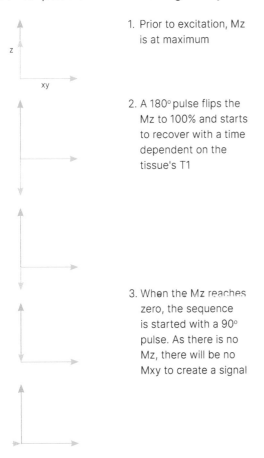

1. Prior to excitation, Mz is at maximum

2. A 180° pulse flips the Mz to 100% and starts to recover with a time dependent on the tissue's T1

3. When the Mz reaches zero, the sequence is started with a 90° pulse. As there is no Mz, there will be no Mxy to create a signal

Figure 161 Time to inversion

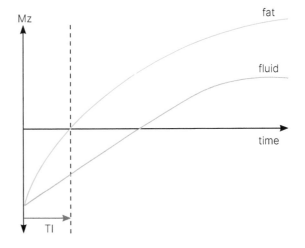

Figure 162 STIR

2) FLAIR (FLuid Attenuated Inversion Recovery)

Fluid signal nulled by selecting long TI (2500 ms)

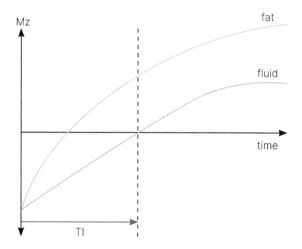

Figure 163 FLAIR

5.15 Diffusion-Weighted Imaging

Diffusion weighted imaging measures the motion of spins (specifically in water). The signal is dependent on the diffusion coefficient within the material i.e. how freely the water can diffuse. The more a particle can move in a given amount of time, the higher the diffusion coefficient.

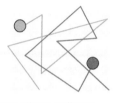

High diffusion coefficient:
Free diffusion particles
e.g. water gel

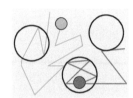

Medium diffusion coefficient:
Free diffusion particles e.g.
normal parenchyma

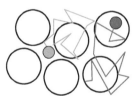

Low diffusion coefficient:
Restricted diffusion due to
many cells e.g. tumours,
abscess

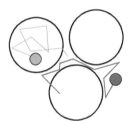

Low diffusion coefficient:
Restricted diffusion due to
swollen cells e.g. infarcts

Figure 164 Diffusion coefficients

Water diffuses randomly via Brownian motion. In pure water and gel, water can diffuse freely with no impediment or restriction. Within soft tissues, water diffusion is impeded by cell membranes and intracellular organelles.

Sequence

A spin-echo sequence is typically used, specifically echo-planar imaging (EPI). EPI minimises the effect of patient motion as it is a very quick sequence. This is important as DWI images the very small motion of water molecules which will be masked by any macroscopic body motion.

Stationary spins
(restricted diffusion)

Mobile spins
(free diffusion)

1. First diffusion gradient applied in a particular direction to dephase the spins.

2. Second diffusion gradient in same direction. This rephases any spins that are still within the gradient field.

Stationary spins return a high signal as they have been exposed to both the dephasing and rephasing gradient.

Mobile spins do not return a signal as they have only been exposed to just one or none of the gradients

Figure 165 Diffusion weighted imaging sequence

Two diffusion gradients are added either side of the 180° RF pulse. The first diffusion gradient dephases the spins. The second diffusion gradient rephases and returns a signal only from the spins that have remained within the area i.e. those that are stationary. Any spins that have moved out of the area aren't rephased and do not return a signal.

The diffusion gradient is applied in multiple directions. The minimum number of directions is 3, running perpendicular to each other (e.g. x-, y-, and z-axes) but, usually, 6-20 directions are used. Each voxel's signal is is an average of the signal from all directions. Then, a standard sequence is run to generate echoes and create the signal.

b-value

The degree of diffusion weighting is represented as the b-value. The more sensitive the DWI sequence is to molecular motion, the higher the b-value.

Higher b-value:
- More sensitive to diffusion
- More noise
- Less signal

Increase the b-value by:
- Larger diffusion gradient (increase the amplitude or the duration)
- Increased time between dephasing and rephasing diffusion gradients

b0 - A DW pulse sequence is first run with the diffusion gradients switched off. This creates a T2*-weighted image that is used for the calculated maps later.

b600-700 - Useful in neonatal brain imaging and body MRI.

b1000 - Strong diffusion weighting. Used to look for cerebral infarcts.

Apparent diffusion coefficient

As DWI images have T2 weighting. Therefore, a lesion that shows as bright on DWI may be bright because of restricted diffusion or because of inherent high T2 signal. The apparent diffusion coefficient (ADC) map is a calculated image that removes the effects of inherent T2 signal.

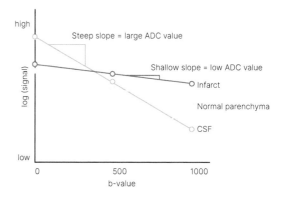

Figure 166 Calculating ADC map

The signal of a tissue decreases exponentially with increasing b-values. If we plot the log of the signal against the b-value, the slope will give us the diffusion characteristics without any T2 signal influence i.e. the ADC signal. Tissues with free diffusion will change signal over different b-values much more than those with restricted diffusion. More diffusion = greater change in signal = a steeper slope = a higher ADC value. This is why restricting lesions will appear dark on the ADC map.

Diffusion Tensor Imaging

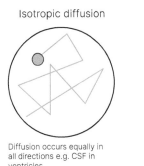
Isotropic diffusion

Diffusion occurs equally in all directions e.g. CSF in ventricles

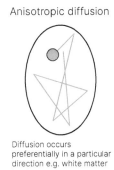
Anisotropic diffusion

Diffusion occurs preferentially in a particular direction e.g. white matter tracts

Figure 167 Isotropic vs anisotrophic diffusion

If the probability of diffusion is the same in every direction, this is called isotropic diffusion e.g. in CSF. Anisotropic diffusion is when diffusion is not equal in every direction e.g. along nerve bundles and white matter tracts. In standard DWI we remove this effect by averaging out the signal obtained from multiple directions. However, we can use this asymmetry in diffusion tensor imaging. The three main techniques are the fractional anisotropy map, the principal diffusion direction map and fibre-tracking maps.

Fractional anisotropy map

Fractional anisotropy (FA) is a measure, from 0 to 1, of the amount of diffusion asymmetry within a voxel. A sphere, which is isotropic, has an FA of 0. The more asymmetric the diffusion becomes the closer FA is to 1. The FA map is gray-scale. The brighter the voxel, the more anisotropic the diffusion.

Principal diffusion direction map

Colours and brightness are assigned to the voxels based on the degree of anisotropy (represented as brightness) and the direction (represented as colours).

Fibre tracking map

The direction of the asymmetry is used to compute fibre trajectories with automated software. A "seed voxel" is selected by the user and the software follows the direction of the adjacent voxels to create an image of the tracts.

Artefacts

T2 shine-through

As the DWI sequence has T2/T2* weighting, high signal on DWI could either be due to restricted diffusion or intrinsic high T2 signal. The ADC map removes the effect of T2 signal. Any region that has low signal on ADC is truly restricting.

T2 dark-through

Just as a lesion with high intrinsic T2 signal will cause T2 shine-through, a lesion with low intrinsic T2 signal will cause low signal on the

DWI, called T2-dark through.

Metal artefact

Because of the T2* weighting of DWI the sequence is very susceptible to anything that disrupts the local magnetic field such as metal or blood products. The region of signal loss around metal can be very large. In the presence of haemorrhage, the signal on DWI is less predictable.

Σ Summary

- DWI sequence
  - Spin echo, usually echo-planar imaging (EPI). Fast so body motion minimised
  - Diffusion gradients either side of 180° pulse
    - Stationary spins (i.e. restricted diffusion) return high signal
    - Mobile spins (i.e. free diffusion) do not return signal
  - Gradients applied in at least 3 different directions
  - Signal in voxel averaged from each direction
- b-value
  - Higher b-value:
    - More sensitive to diffusion
    - More noise
    - Less signal

- Increase b-value by:
    - Larger diffusion gradient (increase amplitude or duration)
    - Increase time between dephasing and rephasing diffusion gradients
  - b0 - sequence run without diffusion gradients. T2*/T2 weighted
  - b600-700 - used in neonatal and body imaging
  - b1000 - used for cerebral infarcts
- Apparent diffusion coefficient (ADC)
  - Log of DWI signals at different b-values plotted. Slope gives ADC signal
  - Removes effect of intrinsic T2 signal
- Diffusion tensor imaging
  - Isotropic diffusion = diffusion same in every direction
  - Anisotropic diffusion = asymmetric diffusion
  - Fractional anisotropy map
    - Measure of asymmetry
    - 0 = isotropic, 1 = extremely anisotropic
    - Grey-scale image
  - Principal diffusion direction map
    - Measures anisotropy and direction
    - Degree of anisotropy = brightness
    - Direction = colour
  - Fibre tracking map
    - Automatic generation of fibre tracks by software
- Artefacts
  - T2 shine-through - intrinsic high T2 signal shows as bright on DWI. ADC removes this effect

- T2 dark-through - intrinsic low T2/T2* signal shows as low signal on DWI
- Metal artefact - DWI very susceptible to artefact created by metal and blood products

5.16 MR Spectroscopy

MR spectroscopy counts as a molecular imaging technique because it can measure the concentration of certain molecules within the imaged region. Different nuclei can be targeted such as carbon-13 and phosphorous-31. However, hydrogen-1 (protons) are the most commonly used due to the high sensitivity of the nuclei, the 100% availability of the isotope and the abundant presence of protons in most metabolites creating a larger signal.

- Advantages of MRS:
    - Can identify concentration of metabolites in imaged tissue
- Disadvantages of MRS:
    - Low resolution
    - Very susceptible to local magnetic field heterogeneity. This is very noticeable when imaging close to bone, calcium and blood. Shimming (homogenisation) of the field can improve artefacts.
    - Can only image limited area

Metabolites

MRS utilises the fact that each metabolite will have a very slightly different Larmor frequency. The frequencies of the returned signals are plotted in units of parts per million (ppm) along with the strength of the signal (i.e. the concentration of the metabolite).

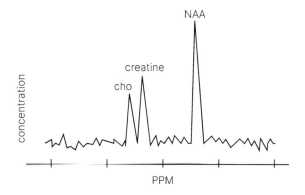

Figure 168 MRS spectrum

The most common metabolites detected and their clinical relevance are outlined below.

	Metabolite	Frequency (ppm)	Role	Clinical relevance
ml	Myoinositol	3,6	Glial marker	Raised in gliomas and MS Reduced in herpetic encephalitis
Cho	Choline	3,2	Cell membrane and metabolism marker	Raised in tumours and demyelination
Cr	Creatine	3,0	Energy metabolism marker	Constant peak
Glx	GABA, glutamine, glutamate	2,1 - 2,5	Intracellular neuronal transmitter	Raised in hepatic encephalopathy

	Metabolite	Frequency (ppm)	Role	Clinical relevance
NAA	N-Acetyl-Aspartate	2,0	Healthy neuronal marker	Raised in Canavan's disease Reduced in any condition resulting in loss of neurons
Lac	Lactate	1,3 doublet	Anaerobic respiration	Raised in ischaemia, seizures, tumours, mitochondrial disorders
Lip	Lipids	0,9 and 1,4		Raised in necrotic tumours
aa	Aminoacids	0,97		Raised in pyogenic abscesses

Performing MRS

1) Voxels

MRS can be single voxel or multivoxel

Single voxel spectroscopy (SVS): a single voxel is selected and analysed.
- Advantages:
  - High signal-to-noise ratio
  - No spectral contamination
  - Short scan times
- Disadvantages:
  - Very small coverage
  - Low resolution

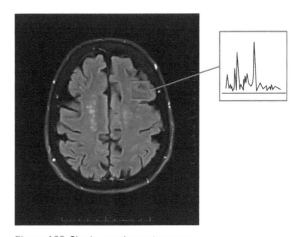

Figure 169 Single voxel spectroscopy

Multi-voxel chemical shift imaging (CSI): multiple voxels in a 1D, 2D or 3D array are selected and a spectrum is produced for each voxel.
- Advantages:
  - Larger total coverage
  - Higher resolution
- Disadvantages:
  - Longer imaging time
  - More likely to have magnetic field inhomogeneities
  - Lower signal-to-noise ratio

- Spectral contamination from adjacent voxels

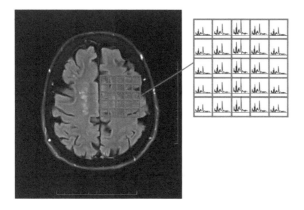

Figure 170 Multi voxel spectroscopy

2) Sequence

1. Suppress water signal

Water contains a large quantity of hydrogen nuclei which masks the small spectroscopic signal from other metabolites. This is usually done with a CHEmical Shift Selective (CHESS) sequence which saturates out the water signal.

2. Select voxel or voxels of interest

With SVS this is done with successive RF pulses in three orthogonal planes which intersect at the voxel of interest. With CSI, phase encoding steps are used to image multiple voxels.

3. Acquire spectrum

Several sequences can be used to acquire the spectrum including Point RESolved Spectroscopy (PRESS) and Stimulated Echo Acquisition Mode (STEAM).

Summary

- MRS utilises different Larmor frequencies based on metabolite composition
- Most often uses protons (^{1}H) but can use ^{13}C or ^{31}P
- Forms spectrum of frequencies present and strength of signal (concentration)
- MRS is low resolution and very susceptible to local magnetic field inhomogeneities

1. Suppress water signal
   - e.g. with CHESS sequence
   - Very high proton count in water masks other weaker signals
2. Select voxel / voxels of interest
   - Single-voxel: quicker, better signal to noise ratio
   - Multi-voxel: better resolution, image larger area
3. Acquire spectrum
   - PRESS and STEAM most common

5.17 MR Angiography

Differences between x-ray, CT and MR angiography:

X-ray	CT	MRI
		Can be contrast enhanced or not. No contrast: Image signal strength due to intrinsic properties of the blood and the flow Contrast: The contrast agent itself is not imaged but the effect it has on the surrounding water
Image signal strength reflects intraluminal density of contrast material - contrast required		
Selective study - contrast injected into specific vessels	Contrast injected intravenously and phase images acquired determines vessels imaged	Non-selective
2D data set	Can obtain 3D data-set	Can obtain 3D data-set

It is first useful to go through some of the flow artefacts created during MR imaging as these are exploited when performing MR angiography.

Flow Effects

1) Time of flight effects

Time of flight effects include:

- Flow-related enhancement
- High-velocity signal loss or "washout"

Flow-related enhancement

Occurs in gradient echo imaging and is a result of **magnetic saturation**

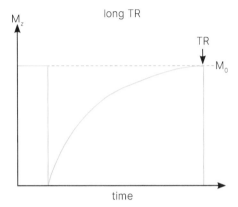

When RF pulse applied (90° in spin echo, <90° in gradient echo) the longitudinal magnetisation (Mz) becomes zero and slowly recovers its longitudinal magnetisation to the initial value (M_0)

Figure 171 Saturation

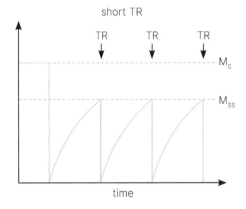

If the RF pulse is re-applied before the Mz has had chance to fully recover, the longitudinal magnetisation never reaches its maximum initial value. The longitudinal magnetisation instead is refigured to a new lower steady state value (M_{ss}). The closer the RF pulses, the less time allowed for Mz to recover, the lower the new M_{ss}.

Figure 172 Saturation 2

Gradient echo involves exposing the tissue to multiple short TRs. Stationary tissue will be subjected to many TRs, reducing the transverse magnetisation. However, fresh blood flowing into the imaging slice will not have been exposed to these TRs and will have a lot more transverse magnetisation than the surrounding tissue. It will, therefore, return a larger signal.

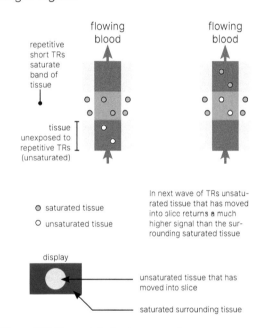

Figure 173 Flow related enhancement

Flow void
Occurs in spin-echo imaging.

The signal from spin echo depends on the tissue receiving both a 90° and 180° RF pulse to generate the echo. If tissue in a slab exposed to the 90° pulse then moves out of the slab it will not receive the 180° RF pulse to be able to generate an echo. Similarly, tissue moving into the slab exposed to the 180° RF pulse will not have been exposed to the 90° RF pulse beforehand.

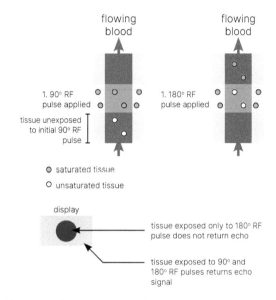

Figure 174 Flow void artefact

The time between the 90 and 180° RF pulses is TE/2. Therefore, if the tissue moves faster than TE/2 all the material exposed to the initial 90° pulse will not be exposed to the 180° pulse. If, however, it moves slightly slower than TE/2, then some material will be exposed to both and generate a small signal, depending upon how much material remains.

2) Spin phase effects

Remember from 5.9 - Phase Encoding that the gradient applied affects the phase of the precessing protons and that magnetic gradients are used to localise the origin of a signal. A proton that is moving along a gradient will alter its phase according the length of time the gradient is applied, the magnitude of the gradient and the velocity of the proton. We know the time and magnitude of the gradient and so we can calculate the velocity of a proton.

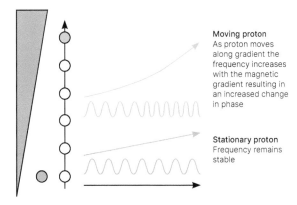

Figure 175 Spin phase effects

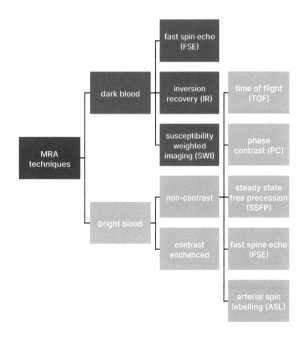

Figure 176 MRA techniques

MR Angiogram Techniques

The types of MR angiograms can be broadly separated out into two types: dark blood and bright blood. The bright blood techniques are then further subdivided according to whether they use gadolinium or not.

The main ones used are time-of-flight, phase contrast and contrast-enhanced techniques.

1) Time of flight (TOF)

This is a **gradient echo** sequence that uses **flow-related enhancement**. It has a short repetition time (TR) to ensure that all stationary spins will have their signal saturated out. Only spins that then move into the imaging field, that have not experienced the saturating RF pulses, will yield a high signal. It can either be a 2D or 3D study.

Pre-saturating bands are used to reduce the signal from blood flowing into the imaging field from a certain direction e.g. apply it distal to the imaging field to saturate out returning venous flow but ensure high signal from outgoing arterial flow.

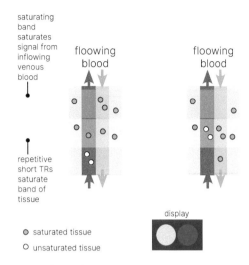

saturating band saturates signal from inflowing venous blood

floowing blood

floowing blood

repetitive short TRs saturate band of tissue

display

○ saturated tissue

○ unsaturated tissue

Figure 177 Saturation band

Advantages

- Contrast agent not required
- Can be used for venous (2D, good for low velocities) or arterial imaging (3D, good for high velocities)
- Very sensitive to flow
- Saturates out all background signal
- 3D TOF is very high resolution (1mm)

Disadvantages

- Flow voids due to:
  - In-plane saturation
  - Post-stenotic turbulence distal to the stenosis
  - Slow flow
- Can exaggerate the length of occlusion and stenosis
- Long imaging time
- Sensitive to metal artefact
- Stationary objects with very high T1 signal will be visible (e.g. haemorrhage)
- Retrograde arterial flow may be obscured

if venous saturation bands have been applied

2) Phase contrast (PC)

Exploits differences in transverse magnetisation i.e. spin phase

Advantages

- Contrast agent not used
- Can reconstruct the data in any plane as usually acquired using 3D method
- Good background suppression
- Insensitive to T1 effects
- Can control the velocity dependent phase shift to alter sensitivity to different flow velocities
- Velocity can be quantificd as well as the direction unlike ToF MRA which is just bright or not

Disadvantages

- Takes 4x as long as TOF as image acquired in three orthogonal directions to create image
- No in-plane flow voids
- More sensitivity to turbulence

3) Contrast enhanced (CE)

Uses Gadolinium Chelate agents which cause shortening of the T1 relaxation of blood compared with background tissue leading to a high signal intensity of blood on T1-weighted sequences. The area of interest is imaged in the first pass of the contrast to ensure the best signal.

Advantages

- More accurate
- Reproducible
- Faster scan so can image at different phases e.g. pre-contrast, arterial, venous
- Fewer flow-related artefacts

Disadvantages

- Not flow-sensitive

5.18 MR Contrast Agents

Magnetism Definitions

Type of magnetism	Definition	Examples
Ferromagnetic	Large magnetic susceptibility i.e. when placed in a magnetic field the field strength is much stronger inside the material than it is outside	Iron Nickel Cobalt
	Remains magnetised when external magnetic field removed	
Superparamagnetic	Consist of some elements of ferromagnetic materials	
	Magnetic susceptibility between ferromagnetic and paramagnetic	
Paramagnetic	Weakly attracted to magnets and, therefore, only weakly influence a magnetic field	Oxygen Magnesium Gadolinium
	Causes T1-shortening and T2-shortening (increases T1 signal intensity, decreases T2 signal intensity)	
Diamagnetic	When placed in a magnetic field will weakly repel the field	Water Copper Nitrogen Barium sulphate
	Results in loss of signal in bowel on MRI after barium sulphate suspensions administered	

Types of Contrast Agents

1) T1 paramagnetic contrast agents

These cause local magnetic field distortions that enhance T1 and T2 relaxation i.e. result in greater T1 signal and lower T2 signal. Factors that affect degree of T1 relaxation:

- Concentration of Gadolinium (Gd) in tissues
- Proximity of surrounding tissues
- Rotational motion of Gd

- Number of water molecules that associate with Gd
- Time that water molecules are around to associate with Gd

The effect of T1 relaxation will increase with the concentration of Gd until an optimum concentration is reached (increasing T1 signal). After this, any further increases in concentration will reduce the T1 signal due to T2 relaxation effects being more prominent. This is why you will sometimes see very low signal within the bladder after gadolinium injection. The contrast has collected to high concentrations and the T2-shortening effect predominates.

Gadolinium

- E.g. gadolinium diethylenetriamine penta-acetic acid (Gd-DTPA), which on its own is toxic so must be encased in another molecule. The different MR contrast agents use different chelates
- Paramagnetic
- T1 contrast agent
- Extracellular
- Allows dynamic phase imaging e.g. arterial, venous and equilibrium

Hepatobiliary agents

- Usually contain manganese
- Paramagnetic
- T1 contrast agent
- Intracellular (taken up by functioning hepatocytes in health liver tissue)
- Agent slowly taken up by hepatocytes
    - Can image up to 24 hours later
    - Doesn't allow for dynamic imaging

2) T2 superparamagnetic contrast agents

The small local magnetic field disruption caused by the contrast agent will slightly alter the precessional frequency of any proton that is in its vicinity. Once the proton moves away it will return to its precessional frequency but with a phase shift (**spin dephasing**) which speeds up the T2 decay and **reduces the T2 signal**.

The higher the concentration of the contrast agent the greater the dephasing and the lower the T2 signal.

Iron oxide

- Superparamagnetic iron oxide (SPIO) and ultrasmall superparamagnetic iron oxide (USPIO) agents
- Superparamagnetic iron oxide does not leak into the interstitium. It remains in the intravascular space until it is eliminated via the reticuloendothelial system
- Coated with substances to increase uptake by the reticuloendothelial system
- Reduces T2 signal of absorbing tissues which decreases the T2 signal
- Requires injection one hour before images acquired

5.19 MR Image Quality

The image quality depends on:

1. Resolution
   - Matrix
   - Field of view (FOV)
   - Slice thickness
2. Signal-to-Noise Ratio (SNR)
3. Contrast
4. Artefacts

Artefacts are covered later in the 5.20 - MR Artefacts section and contrast depends on the scan parameters.

Resolution

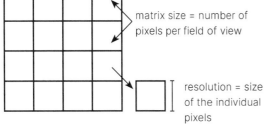

field of view – size of the area being imaged

matrix size = number of pixels per field of view

resolution = size of the individual pixels

Figure 178 Matrix

The resolution is the size of the individual pixel (2D) or voxel (3D). The smaller the pixel or voxel the greater the resolution. It is intimately related to the field of view, the matrix size and the slice thickness as shown in the equation below.

$$\text{Pixel area} = \text{field of view} / \text{matrix}$$

$$\text{Voxel volume} = (\text{field of view} / \text{matrix}) \times \text{slice thickness}$$

1) Matrix

The matrix size is the number of pixels in the image. Increasing the matrix size will increase the number of pixels in the image but, as they are still within the same **field of view**, they will be smaller.

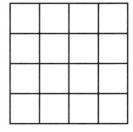

matrix size: 4 × 4 = 16
FOV: 4 × 4 mm = 16 mm
resolution: 1 mm
(4 mm / 4 voxels)

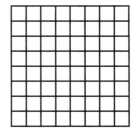

matrix size: 8 × 8 = 64
FOV: 4 × 4 mm = 16 mm
resolution: 0.5 mm
(4 mm / 8 voxels)

Figure 179 Matrix size

Increasing the matrix size:

- Increases spatial resolution - smaller pixels/voxels means better detail
- Decreases signal - there are fewer photons per voxel so the signal is less
- Increases scan time - more voxels need to be acquired (note this is only in the phase encoding direction as each voxel requires a new signal) i.e. more voxels means more signals need to be created.

2) Field of view

matrix size: 4 × 4 = 16
FOV: 4 × 4 mm = 16 mm
resolution: 1 mm
(4 mm / 4 voxels)

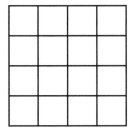

matrix size: 4 × 4 = 16
FOV: 6 × 6 mm = 64 mm
resolution: 1.5 mm
(6 mm / 4 voxels)

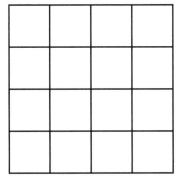

Figure 180 Matrix - field of view

The field of view (FOV) determines the size of the area to be imaged; a larger field of view means a larger area imaged. The matrix size remains the same and so, to fill up a larger area, the voxel becomes larger.

Increasing the FOV:
- Increases the signal - a larger voxel means more signal received per voxel
- Lower resolution - the voxels become larger
- Increased viewing area

3) Slice thickness

Increasing the slice thickness:
- Increases the signal
- Decreases the resolution
- Increases the partial volume effect
- Gives larger object coverage

Slice Gap

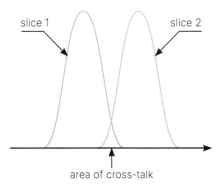

Figure 181 Slice thickness

The slice gap is the amount of space between slices. It is measured as a percentage of the slice thickness. In the real world, slices are not perfect and the signals form a bell-shaped curve. The slice gap is the gap between the peaks of these curves. We want to minimise the amount of space between each slice to prevent sections being missed. However, when slices overlap an area of **cross-talk** results which causes artefacts (the overlapping area contains signal from both slices and the protons become saturated resulting in no signal). Usually, a gap of 10-20% is used to minimise the cross talk

Increased slice gap:
- Less cross-talk
- Increased coverage - slices placed further apart and, therefore, cover a larger area.

Another way to avoid cross-talk artefact is to image non-contiguous slices (e.g. slices 1, 3 and 5 in one sequence and then 2, 4 and 6).

Signal-to-Noise Ratio

The signal-to-noise ratio (SNR) is a useful concept in every modality of radiology. There is always background noise in x-ray, CT and MRI. To get a useful picture, the amount of signal from the thing being imaged should be greater than the noise. A higher SNR means a better and more useful image (more signal than there is noise).

The greater the size of the voxel / pixel the more signal there is per point in the image, improving the SNR. However, a greater voxel / pixel means each point in the image is larger and the resolution is lower.

Higher resolution = lower SNR (assuming all other factors remain equal)

4) Number of Acquisitions

Another way to improve the signal is to scan the same area several times. This is determined by the number of acquisitions (Number of Signal Averages (NEX/NSA)). Each acquisition fills k-space. We can repeat the number of acquisitions and then average the signals to create the image, thus collecting more signal per slice imaged.

Increasing NEX:
- Increases signal - however, the signal is only increased by √NEX (doubling the NEX only increases the SNR by √2 i.e. 1.4)
- Less noise
- Fewer artefacts due to signal averaging
- Increased scan time - doubling the NEX doubles the scan time

Summary

- Pixel area = field of view / matrix
- Voxel volume = (field of view / matrix) x slice thickness

- Increasing the matrix size:
  - Increases spatial resolution
  - Decreases signal
  - Increases scan time
- Increasing the FOV:
  - Increases the signal
  - Lower resolution
  - Increased viewing area
- Increasing the slice thickness:
  - Increases the signal
  - Decreases the resolution
  - Increases the partial volume effect
  - Gives larger object coverage
- Increased slice gap:
  - Less cross-talk
  - Increased coverage
- Increasing NEX:
  - Increases signal
  - Less noise
  - Fewer artefacts due to signal averaging
  - Increased scan time
- To improve the SNR:
  - Increase NEX
  - Lower resolution
  - Thicker slices
  - Larger FOV
  - Use surface coils
- To improve the resolution:
  - Increase the matrix
  - Decrease the FOV
  - Decrease the slice thickness

5.20 MR Artefacts

Motion Artefacts

1) Patient motion

- e.g. patient moving during scan, cardiac motion, breathing
- Effect:
  - Ghosting: low intensity copies of the original image are shifted in the **phase-encoding** direction
- Solutions:
  - Acquire more signals
  - Image with very fast single shot sequences
  - Change phase and frequency directions during the scan
  - ECG gating for cardiac motion artefacts
  - Breath-hold scanning for breathing artefacts
  - Navigator echo triggering for breathing artefacts: triggers scan only when boundary between lung and liver is within a certain acceptance window

2) Flow artefacts

(See 5.17 - MR Angiography section for more information)

Distortion artefacts

- Due to inhomogeneities in the magnetic field:
  - Local field inhomogeneity
  - Non-linearities in gradient magnetic fields
  - Boundaries between tissues of different magnetic susceptibilities

1) Local field inhomogeneity

The local field is most commonly distorted by metal present in the object which causes two types of artefacts: signal loss due to dephasing and distortion. An air-fluid interface can also cause similar inhomogeneities.

- Dephasing of transverse magnetisation
  - Interferes with T2 transverse magnetisation so it dephases much quicker and doesn't return an echo
- Distortion
  - Local field inhomogeneities affect the magnetic field gradient and, therefore, the Larmor frequency
  - As location is encoded based on Larmor frequency this leads to protons in the area of the inhomogeneity being encoded in the incorrect position

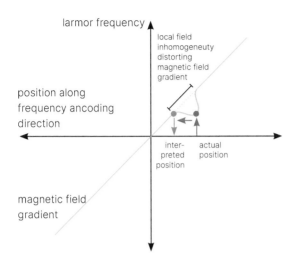

Figure 182 Metal artefact

2) Non-linearities in magnetic field gradient

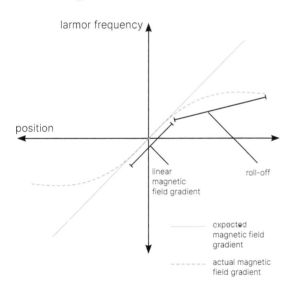

Figure 183 Non-linear gradient

The gradients used in spatial encoding are meant to be linear but often they roll off from the straight line towards the edges of the FOV. The distortion created occurs in both the **frequency- and phase-encoding** directions.

Solution:

- Correction often made automatically as the non-linearities are known and can be adjusted for.

3) Boundaries between tissues

The most common two substances in the human body are water and fat. Protons in water and fat will resonate at slightly different Larmor frequencies despite being in the same position in the magnetic field gradients. There are two artefacts that are produced by this property when protons from these two tissues are in close proximity: chemical-shift and fat/water cancellation.

Chemical shift

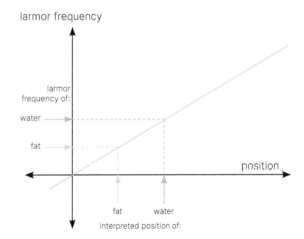

Figure 184 Chemical shift artefact

Protons in fat and water resonate at slightly different Larmor frequencies. This means that even when they exist in the same position they will be interpreted as being in slightly different positions in the **frequency-encoding** direction which uses the precessing frequency to encode position.

Fat/water cancellation

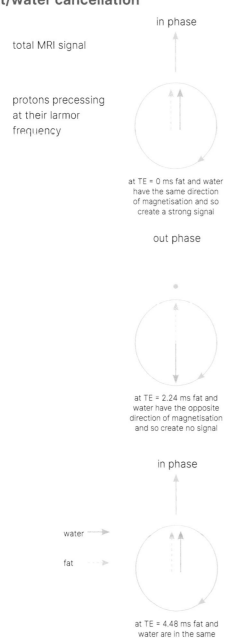

total MRI signal

in phase

protons precessing at their larmor frequency

at TE = 0 ms fat and water have the same direction of magnetisation and so create a strong signal

out phase

at TE = 2.24 ms fat and water have the opposite direction of magnetisation and so create no signal

in phase

water

fat

at TE = 4.48 ms fat and water are in the same direction again

Figure 185 Fat cancellation

As protons from fat and water have different Larmor frequencies they will go in and out of phase over time. If a voxel contains both fat and water the signals from the two may cancel each other out if the TE of a certain length is used (2.24 ms at 1.5 T). This creates a signal loss with a black line between tissues that contain both fat and water.

This is used in liver MRI out-of-phase imaging as fatty infiltration results in cancelling of the signal helping with diagnosis.

Note:
- Chemical shift is from boundaries between fat and water (i.e. macroscopic)
- Fat/water cancellation nulls the signal from microscopic fat (i.e. fat and water present in the same voxel)
- Fat saturation imaging cancels signal from macroscopic fat (i.e. fat and water present in different voxels)

Fat Saturation Artefact

Fat saturation (see 5.14 - Inversion Recovery Sequences) imaging exploits the different Larmor frequencies of fat and water by applying a narrow RF pulse centred over the fat peak that nulls the signal. If the frequency of the fat peak is slightly different - most commonly due to anatomy with a rapidly changing contour (e.g. ankle and foot) or non-linearity of the magnetic field gradient at the periphery of the image as explained earlier - the RF pulse will not be positioned over the fat peak any more and will fail to null the signal.

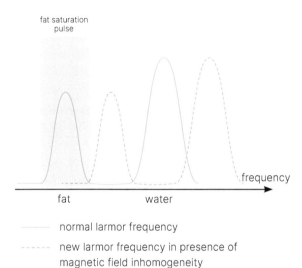

Figure 186 Failure of fat saturation

Radiofrequency Artefacts

1) Improper coil selection

RF coil elements can be switched on and off depending on the FOV required.
- RF coil in FOV switched off = loss of signal in this area
- RF coil outside FOV switched on = artefacts such as ghosting from motion being aliased back onto the FOV

2) Spurious RF signals

RF signals arising from outside due to an inadequately shielded MRI room or inside from faulty equipment will contribute to the image. A band of noise will appear in the image in the **phase-encoding direction** depending upon the frequency/frequencies of the external RF signal.

Data Collection Artefacts

1) Inadequate FOV

Signal from structures that lie outside the FOV in the phase encoding direction will be aliased back onto the image (aka **phase wrap**).

Solution:
- Adequate FOV in phase-encoding direction
- If small FOV required can use over-sampling

2) Spurious data

Any spurious data will be encoded into the k-space data as a wave which is encoded into the final image as a **"herringbone"** artefact with alternating light and dark bands.

Sources of spurious data:

- Malfunctioning equipment in scanner room
- Static build-up on clothing

3) Edge representation

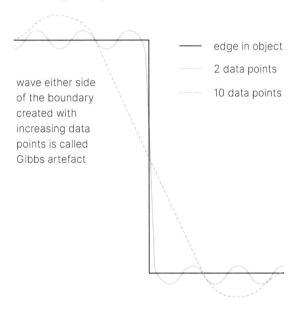

edge in object

2 data points

10 data points

wave either side of the boundary created with increasing data points is called Gibbs artefact

Figure 187 Gibbs artefact

Imaging an edge boundary can create a **Gibbs** or **edge ringing artefact**. The more data points that are acquired the better the boundary edges are represented. However, at the edges of the image the extra data points create superimposed waves which are encoded into the image. This is of particular importance in imaging the spine in which encoding the edge boundary between the spinal cord and CSF can create artefactual lesions within the cord.

Sequence Specific Artefacts

1) Echo-planar imaging (EPI)

Local magnetic field inhomogeneity distortion

In EPI the whole of the k-space is acquired in one RF excitation resulting in very rapid imaging. The horizontal acquisition is very quick but the vertical acquisition is slower. This difference leads to distortion, especially where there are small local magnetic field inhomogeneities such as around the nasal cavity or the orbits.

Solution:
- Parallel or multi-shot EPI: k-space acquired in more than one shot but each shot is faster

N/2 ghosts

A low intensity copy of the image which is shifted by half the FOV in the **phase encoding direction** can occur which is due to misalignment of echoes as the k-space is acquired back and forth.

Solution:
- Careful gradient calibrations

2) Fast spin echo (FSE)

Multiple lines of the k-space are acquired after a signal RF excitation as explained in 5.12 - Spin Echo Sequences - Detailed. The number of lines acquired per TR (or **echo-train length, ETL**) can be very long to the point that the whole of k-space is acquired in a single TR (single-shot FSE). However, over time there will be T2 relaxation that will cause blurring in the image in the **phase encoding direction**.

3) Steady state free precession (SSFP)

In SSFP imaging if there are local magnetic field inhomogeneities this can produce a banding pattern on the image with signal void and stimulated-echoes that constructively and destructively interfere.

5.21 MR Safety

There are multiple national and international bodies that regulate MRI exposure doses for patients, volunteers and staff.

- Medicines and Healthcare Products Regulatory Agency (MHRA) for the use of MRI in patients and the exposure of staff.
- International Electrotechnical Commission (IEC) (2010): provides standards for manufacturers of medical MRI equipment to follow
- International Commission on Non-Ionizing Radiation Protection (ICNIRP): guidance for occupational and general public exposure.

The limits are specific to different modes of scanning. These are:

- Routine / normal operating mode: normal patient studies
- Specific / controlled operating mode: specific studies outside of the normal operating mode. Patient must have panic button with free verbal contact and constant visual contact
- Research / experimental operating mode: examinations conducted at levels above controlled operating mode. These require approval by an ethic committee.

MR Safety Marking

MR Safe	"an item that poses no known hazards resulting from exposures to any MR environment. MR Safe items are composed of materials that are electrically nonconductive, nonmetallic, and nonmagnetic"*
MR Conditional	"an item with demonstrated safety in the MR environment within defined conditions."*
MR Unsafe	"an item that poses unacceptable risks to the patient, medical staff or other persons within the MR environment."*

* Definitions from the ASTM international standard F2503-13

Static Magnetic Field

1) MHRA guideline for whole body exposure of patients

Mode	Tesla
Normal	4.0
Controlled	8.0
Research	No limit
Pregnant	< 2.5

Staff - MHRA guideline for exposure of staff
< 2T for whole body
< 5T for limbs
Over 24h average exposure should not exceed 0.2T

2) Controlled area

5 Gauss line (0.5 mT) is drawn around the room in which the static magnetic power is greater than or equal to 5 Gauss. Patients / staff with contraindications (pacemakers etc.) to MRI should not enter this area.

Radiofrequency (RF) Fields

RF fields cause microwave heating. This is due to the oscillating electromagnetic fields creating electrical currents in patient tissues that then produces heat.

Specific absorption ratio (SAR) = RF energy deposited per mass of tissue (Watts / kg).

1 SAR = 1 W/kg = whole body temperature rise of 0.5 degrees

1) Legislation

Current recommendations are set by the International Committee on Non-ionising Radiation Protection (ICNIRP) (2014).

Whole body exposure:
For whole-body exposures the patient temperature should not increase by **more than 1°c** during an examination.

For infants, pregnant women, and those with cardiocirculatory impairment the temperature increase should not exceed **0.5°c**.

Local exposure:

Localised temperature limits

Operating mode	Head (°c)	Trunk (°c)	Extremities (°c)	SAR (W/kg)
Normal	38	39	40	2
Controlled	38	39	40	4
Restricted	39	40	41	> 4

- **Normal operating mode:** output values do not cause physiological stress to patients. Default SAR is 2 W/Kg.
- **Controlled operating mode:** one or more more outputs may reach a value that may cause physiological stress to patients. These studies need to have medical supervision. Default SAR is 4 W/Kg.
- **Restricted operating mode:** one or more output values may produce significant risk for patients. These studies require explicit ethical approval. SAR is > 4 W/Kg.

2) Factors that affect SAR

The risk of a rise in body temperature is increased in certain patients:
- Patients who are unable to thermoregulate adequately (e.g. heart failure, fever, pregnancy (risk of fetal heating), patients taking medication that affects thermoregulation

(vasodilators, tranquilisers and diuretics)

- Patients in a cast
- Patients who are unable to communicate any heat sensations

Higher SAR	Lower SAR
Large body parts	Small body parts
High static fields (higher Tesla. Doubling the magnetic field from 1.5 T to 3 T leads to a 4x increase in SAR)	Low static fields
180° RF pulse	90° RF pulse
Spin echo: large RF pulses applied very rapidly means higher deposition of energy	Gradient echo: smaller RF pulses. Although these are also applied rapidly the net deposition of energy is lower than in spin echo
Time-of-flight MRA: although this is a gradient echo the RF pulses are applied at a very high speed	
High conductivity tissues (blood, brain, liver, CSF)	Low conductivity tissue (bone marrow, fat)

3) Techniques to reduce SAR

- Increase the TR (apply the RF pulses less rapidly)
- Reduce the flip angle
- Reduce the number of slices in each acquisition
- Reduce the number of echoes in multiecho sequences
- Reduce room temperature and dress patients in light clothing
- Alternate high and low SAR sequences

Gradient Fields

1) ICNIRP and MHRA Limits for exposure to patients

- **Normal operating mode:** 80% of median perception threshold
- **Controlled operating mode:** 100% of median operating
- **Research operating mode:** none available but suggested limit of 120% of median perception threshold

2) Induced currents and voltages

These time-varying gradient fields cause eddying currents in conductive tissues and cause **stimulation** e.g.:
- Peripheral nerve stimulation
- Involuntary muscular contraction
- Breathing difficulties
- Ventricular fibrillation

For static fields greater than 3T:
- Flashes of light on the retina
- Vertigo
- Nausea
- Sensation of metallic taste

The voltages induced may also affect devices:
- Cardiac pacemakers
- Cochlear implants
- ECG monitors

- The fast-switching magnetic fields in gradient echo sequences create loud noises.
- Louder noise caused by:
  - Higher field strength
  - Higher gradient amplitudes
- Machine limit is 140 dB (most don't exceed 120 dB)
- Hearing protection needed to prevent irreversible damage at 90 dB

Metal Related Hazards

1) Ferromagnetic missile effect

- Caused by static field
- At 1.5T, objects can reach an acceleration 10x that of gravity and can reach speeds of >80 k/h once they reach the centre of the bore, usually where the patient's head is positioned

2) Migration / rotation of metal in body

- Caused by static field
- May cause ferromagnetic metal containing objects to migrate within the body or rotate to align with the field like the needle of a compass.
- Of particular concern near the eye or ear e.g. shrapnel in the eye causing sub-retinal haemorrhage and blindness

3) Heating of metal objects

- Caused by RF wave
- Thought to be due to **resonant antenna effect**. RF pulses set up a standing voltage wave in the metal causing tips of wires to undergo rapid heating and burn the patient
- Pacemaker forms conductive circuit
  - RF pulse may induce pulses that cause heart to contract
  - Resonant antenna effect may cause heating up of wires
- Solutions:
  - MR compatible leads
  - Place ECG electrodes as close together as possible to minimise area of conductive loop formed
  - Braid cables
  - Keep cables close to the centre (area of lowest fields)

Contraindications

1) Absolute

- Pacemaker / defibrillator that is non-MRI compatible
- Metallic foreign body in the eye
- Deep brain stimulator
- Bullets or gunshot pellets

- Cerebral aneurysm clips that are non-MRI compatible
- Cochlear implant
- Drug infusion device - might malfunction

2) Relative

- Surgical clips, wire sutures etc
- Joint replacement or prosthesis
- Large patients might not fit into scanner
- Claustrophobic patient
- Significant pain or other conditions that might limit patient's ability to sit still
- Surgery in previous 6 weeks
- Pregnancy - usually not performed in first trimester

Emergencies

1) Cardiac Arrest

- Patient is removed from the magnet on to an MR-compatible trolley and taken outside the controlled area
- Here, resuscitation can commence
- Appliances such as oxygen cylinders must not be brought to the patient in the scanner due to the ferromagnetic missile effect

2) Fire

- Non-ferrous carbon dioxide extinguishers should be used
- Fire-fighting equipment should be used only at a distance of 1m or more from the bore
- If fire-fighters definitely need access to the room the magnet must be quenched to switch it off

3) Quench

- If the magnet has to be switched off e.g.:
  - Person caught between a metal object and the machine
  - Fire
- Quenching the machine involves converting 1000+ litres of liquid helium (which is necessary to cool the magnet) into gascous helium
- This is a very quick event and the gas needs to be vented out into the atmosphere as quickly as possible
- A quench can cost £10,000 worth of lost helium
- Helium displaces oxygen and so oxygen monitors are used and staff should be evacuated from the whole MR suite as asphyxiation can occur

Summary

- MHRA guideline for **patient** whole body exposure
  - Normal < 4T

- Controlled 8T
- Research > no limit (needs approval by Ethics committee)
- Pregnant < 2T (usually avoided in first trimester)
- Guideline for **staff** exposure
  - < 2T for whole body
  - < 5T for limbs
  - Should not exceed 0.2T over 24h
- Controlled area
  - Where stray field is greater than or equal to 5 Gauss (0.5 mT)
  - Patients / staff with contraindications to MR are excluded from this area
- Radiofrequency Fields
  - Cause microwave heating
  - **Measured by** Specific Absorption Ratio (SAR) **= Watts / kg**
  - 1 W/kg = temperature rise of 0.5 °c
- Gradient Fields
  - Induced currents and voltages - cause stimulation of peripheral nerves, muscles and possible ventricular fibrillation
  - Acoustic noise - maximum machine allowance is 140 dB
- Metal Related Hazards
  - Ferromagnetic missile effect - caused by static magnetic field
  - Migration / rotation of metal in body - caused by static magnetic field
  - Heating of metal objects - caused by RF wave
- Contraindications
  - Absolute
    - Non-MR compatible pacemaker / cochlear implant
    - Metallic foreign body in eye
    - Bullets
    - Non-MR compatible cerebral aneurysm clips
  - Relative
    - Surgical clips
    - Surgery in previous 6 weeks
    - Joint replacement / prosthesis
    - Claustrophobic
    - Large patient
    - Inability to lie still
    - Pregnancy - not scanned in first trimester usually

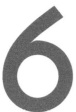

Whereas CT and plain radiographs can only assess the physical structure of the object being imaged, molecular imaging assesses the physiology at a molecular and cellular level. Molecular imaging can be nuclear, using radiopharmaceuticals, or non-nuclear and nuclear imaging can be in vivo or in vitro. Additionally, nuclear medicine is the field of using radiopharmaceuticals to measure and image physiological functions and to treat conditions, such as hyperthyroidism.

This chapter will focus on nuclear imaging and covers radiopharmaceuticals, gamma camera imaging, planar imaging, SPECT, PET, factors affecting image quality, artefacts and quality assurance in nuclear imaging.

6.1	Introduction to Molecular Imaging	211
6.2	Non-Nuclear Molecular Imaging	212
6.3	Production of Radioisotopes	215
6.4	Radiopharmaceuticals	219
6.5	Gamma Camera	225
6.6	Planar Imaging	232
6.7	SPECT Imaging	236
6.8	PET Imaging	240
6.9	NM Image Quality	246
6.10	NM Artefacts	252
6.11	NM Quality Assurance	254

6.1 Introduction to Molecular Imaging

Molecular imaging is the process in which a substance that binds to a target molecule, e.g. a receptor, can be used to image and measure physiological functions in the human body. It is generally separated into non-nuclear and nuclear imaging and nuclear imaging is further separated out into in vivo and in vitro imaging.

In vivo: this is when the tracer radioactivity is measured as it leaves the human body. Radionuclide imaging is an example of this in which a radiopharmaceutical is introduced into the patient and then a gamma camera images the radioactivity leaving the patient (e.g. bone scans)

In vitro: this is when a tracer is introduced into the patient and then tissue / fluid samples taken from the patient and the radioactivity measured from these. No images are produced.

This chapter will focus mostly on nuclear, aka radionuclide, imaging. Nuclear imaging involves the introduction of a radioactive source into the patient. This is done with radiopharmaceuticals which consist of a **radionuclide** that emits gamma radiation and a **pharmaceutical** part which is the physical/chemical component to which the radionuclide is attached to. It is the pharmaceutical that largely determines the physiological behaviour of the radiopharmaceutical and, therefore, the nature of the image obtained.

6.2 Non-Nuclear Molecular Imaging

Non-nuclear molecular imaging consists of techniques that assess the cellular and physiological behaviour without using radioactive materials. These include:

- Contrast-enhanced ultrasound
- Optical imaging
- Magnetic resonance spectroscopy. This is covered in 5.16 - MR Spectroscopy.

Contrast-Enhanced Ultrasound

Contrast-enhanced ultrasound (CEUS) involves the injection of microbubbles. Microbubbles are structures measuring 1 to 4 μm formed of a high-molecular-weight gas core, such as perfluorocarbons and sulphur hexafluoride, with a shell typically made of lipid. After injection, they circulate in the blood for a few minutes until they are removed by the reticuloendothelial system or are broken down naturally or by the ultrasound wave.

They are highly echogenic due to the impedance mismatch between the gas and blood / tissue. This non-targetted technique has been used to assess blood flow (e.g. in patent foramen ovale) and perfusion (e.g. liver tumours).

CEUS in molecular imaging

More recently, ligands are being added to the shells to turn them into molecular imaging agents i.e. they will bind to specific molecular targets. As the ultrasound bubbles are relatively large they are limited to vascular targets. The current targets undergoing research are angiogenesis markers (e.g. VEGF), inflammatory markers (e.g. ICAM-1) and thrombosis markers (e.g. GPIIb-IIIa).

Although CEUS is in common use clinically, targeted CEUS in which ligands have been added to the shell of the bubbles is still in the pre-clinical stages.

Advantages:
- No radiation
- Rapid acquisition of images
- Real-time scanning
- Simple equipment

Disadvantages:
- Microbubbles are short-lived
- Can only scan small areas
- Very operator dependent

Optical imaging

Optical imaging utilises processes that produce visible photons that can then be detected and measured. The two main techniques are bioluminescence and fluorescence.

Advantages:
- No radiation
- In fluorescence the signal can be repeatedly obtained
- Rapid acquisition of images
- Real-time imaging

Disadvantages:
- Low background signal
- Scatter of released photons
- Limited depth of penetration of the photons i.e. only suitable for superficial structures

1) Bioluminescence

Bioluminescence imaging utilises biochemical reaction of the enzyme luciferase in which optical photons are created. Luciferin is injected and, when it enters a cell containing the enzyme luciferase, a chemical reaction occurs in which a detectable photon is produced. Cells that typically contain luciferase are tumour cells making bioluminescence useful for detecting the presence of tumour cells and response to therapy.

2) Fluorescence

In fluorescence the injected molecule is activated with an external light source of appropriate wavelength and then the photon emissions released from the decay of the excited state are measured. The advantage of fluorescence is that the molecules can be repeatedly excited (to a limit) to keep measuring a signal.

Summary

- Non-nuclear molecular imaging consists of:
  - Molecular targeted imaging without the use of radiation
- Contrast-enhanced ultrasound
  - Microbubbles 1-4 µm filled with perfluorocarbons and sulphur hexafluoride with a lipid shell
  - Research into attaching ligands to shells for molecular targeting
  - Advantages: quick, easy to use equipment, real-time
  - Disadvantages: very operator dependent, can only scan small areas, microbubbles short-lived
- Optical imaging
  - Detectable photons released which create the image
  - Two types:
    - Bioluminescence: luciferin injected which is broken down by luciferase enzyme in cancer cells and releases detectable photons
    - Fluorescence: Molecules activated with light and release detectable photons with the excitable state decays

- Advantages: quick, real-time imaging, in fluorescence molecules can be repeatedly excited
- Disadvantages: low background signal, limited depth of penetration of released photons, photons scatter
- MR spectroscopy
  - Covered in 5.16 MR Spectroscopy.

6.3 Production of Radioisotopes

There are three methods for producing radioisotopes:

- Cyclotron
- Nuclear reactor
- Radionuclide generator

1) Cyclotron

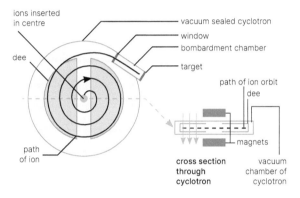

Figure 188 Cyclotron

This method of producing radioisotopes is also called nuclear bombardment.

1. The cyclotron consists of a vacuum chamber into which particles are injected into the centre
2. These are accelerated in a circular path by a high frequency alternating voltage applied between two D-shaped electrodes (these are called "dee's"). The dee's are hollow and allow the particles to move between them
3. The particles are then made to move in a spiral pattern from the centre of the vacuum chamber to the outside by applying a large static magnetic field

4. As the particles' path leads them to the edge of the cyclotron they eventually enter the bombardment chamber and interact with the target to produce the radioisotopes.

Cyclotron produced radioisotopes

- Technetium-99m - used in 80% of nuclear medicine studies. The target is molybdenum which is bombarded to produce molybdenum-99. This then decays to Technetium-99m which is used in imaging.
- Fluorine-18 - used in FDG PET scanning as well as with choline. Created by bombarding ^{18}O rich water with protons to produce ^{18}F. ^{18}F has a half-life of 1.87 hours and releases gamma rays with an energy of 511 keV.
- Gallium-67 - used as ^{67}Ga-citrate for imaging of inflammation / tumours.
- Thallium-201 - used as ^{201}Tl-chloride in cardiac function imaging.

2) Nuclear reactor

1. The core of ^{235}Uranium undergoes spontaneous fission into lighter fragments emitting two or three fission neutrons in the process
2. These fission neutrons then interact with ^{235}U to produce the highly unstable ^{236}U which carries on the fission event in a

self-sustaining nuclear chain reaction

3. Materials can be lowered into ports in the reactor to be irradiated by the neutrons. Neutron capture then creates isotopes of the target element

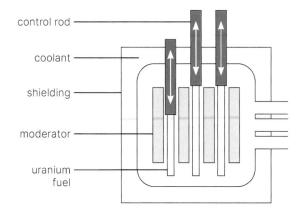

Figure 189 Nuclear generator

The fission activity can be controlled with control rods that engulf the cores and are made of material that absorbs the neutrons without undergoing fission (e.g. cadmium or boron) preventing further fission events.

The moderator rods are made of a material that slows down the energetic fission neutrons. Slower neutrons are more efficient at initiating additional fission events.

Radionuclides produced by neutron activation

- Neutrons are added to isotopes creating a heavy isotope that generally lie above the line of stability. This means they tend to decay in β-emission.
- Only a very small fraction of the target nuclei are activated

- A disadvantage of a nuclear reactor is the relatively low yield of the desired radioisotope and the substantial production of other radioisotopes.

Reactor produced radioisotopes

- Molybdenum-98 - used in cyclotrons to produce molybenum-99 which decays to technetium-99m
- Iodine-131 - used in treating and in imaging the thyroid gland
- Xenon-133 - used in lung ventilation studies. Half-life of 5 days so can be transported readily unlike krypton-81m (half-life of 13 seconds)

3) Radionuclide generator

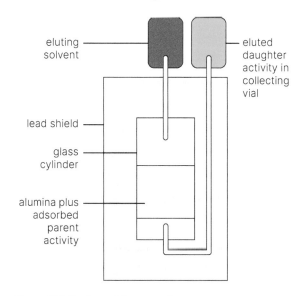

Figure 190 Radionuclide generator

1. A slow-decaying parent radionuclide is adsorbed onto a surface such as alumina in a sterile glass column encased in a lead

or depleted uranium shield

2. This parent radionuclide decays into the shorter-lived radionuclide that will be used for the nuclear imaging - the "daughter" radionuclide
3. The "daughter" radionuclide is removed by passing an eluting solvent (such as sterile saline) through the glass column
4. The resulting solution is collected into a vial which collects the daughter solvent via a vacuum action

This method of producing radionuclides is useful when using a short lived radionuclide as it needs to be produced near the patient. In this way the generator can travel whilst producing the daughter radioisotope to the site of use at which point it can be eluted. Each time the radioisotope is eluted its activity (concentration) drops to zero. It then steadily builds up again until it is eluted again.

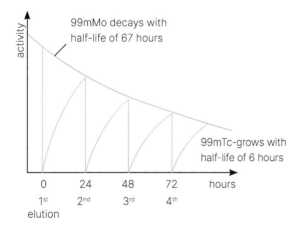

Figure 191 Decay in a generator

Generator produced radionuclides

Technetium-99m, the most commonly used radioisotope, is produced in this way from the longer-lived Molybdenum-99 (created by cyclotrons) which decays via beta decay.

Another radioisotope produced by this method is Krypton-81m, used in lung ventilation studies.

▪ Rubidium-81 is produced by a cyclotron
▪ Adsorbed onto zirconium phosphate in the generator
▪ Decays into Krypton-81m by electron capture and beta decay
▪ Krypton-81m is then extracted from the column by blowing air through it

Summary

Cyclotron

1. Particles injected into centre
2. Accelerated in spiral path to the outside by Dee electrodes and static magnetic field
3. Enter bombardment chamber and interact with target to produce radioisotopes
▪ Products: Fluorine-18, Gallium-67, Thalium-201, Krypton-81m, Molybdenum-99

Nuclear reactor

1. Core Uranium-235 undergoes spontaneous fission releasing neutrons
2. Neutrons interact with Uranium-235 releasing highly unstable Uranium-236

which induces further fission - chain re-action

3. Materials lowered into ports to be irradiated by neutrons and converting into desired isotope

- Fission activity controlled by control rods that cover uranium rods and absorb fission neutrons to prevent a chain reaction

- Moderator rods slow down energetic fission neutrons to make fission more efficient

- Products: Molybdenum, Iodine-131, Xenon-133

Generator

1. Parent radionuclide adsorbed onto surface e.g alumina in a glass column. Decays into daughter nuclide

2. Daughter nuclide removed by passing solvent through the glass column

3. Eluted daughter activity collected in vial via vacuum action

- Products: Technetium-99m, Krypton-81m

6.4 Radiopharmaceuticals

Radiopharmaceuticals consist of a radioactive isotope, which creates the image, and a pharmaceutical, which determines the physiological behaviour of the compound and, therefore, where the signal accumulates to form the image.

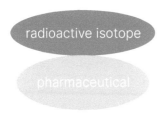

Figure 192 Radiopharmaceutical

There are several properties of the ideal radioisotope for diagnostic purposes (i.e. not therapeutic):

- Half life which is short enough to limit radiation dose to patient but long enough to allow good signal during imaging (ideally 1.5 x length of imaging)
- Emits gamma rays which are of high enough energy to leave the body, reach the camera and contribute to the image. The low energy of alpha or beta particles means they are absorbed by the body which increases the radiation dose to the patient and limits the radiation that reaches the camera to produce the image
- Mono-energetic gamma emitter (i.e. gamma rays of one energy). The ideal energy range is 100 to 250 keV for optimal imaging
- Decays to stable daughter isotopes that will not cause significant radiation dose to patient
- Easy to bind to different pharmaceuticals
- Doesn't change behaviour of pharmaceutical

And there are several properties of the ideal pharmaceutical:

- High target:non-target uptake ratio
- Easy and cheap to produce
- Non-toxic
- Does not alter physiology in order to give accurate depiction of patient's physiology

Clinical Radiopharmaceuticals

There are many combinations of radioisotopes and pharmaceuticals that are used in medicine and in imaging. Some of these will produce an image and other will just produce a measurement but no image.

1) Classification by system

The most common imaging tests for different systems have been outlined below.

Cardiac imaging

- **Thallium-201:** For myocardial perfusion. Injected while the patient is in peak exercise or shortly after the pharmacological stress agent (adenosine) is administered. Patient is imaged immediately to see muscle that is non-perfused and then 3-4 hours later to see muscle that is persistently non-perfused i.e. irreversible infarct vs. poorly perfused i.e. ischaemia.

- **Technetium-99m (99mTc) sestamibi or tetrofosmin:** For myocardial perfusion. This has a shorter half-life than thallium-201. It also requires a second injection on the delayed study.
- **MUGA:** For ventriculography. The patient's RBCs are radiolabelled and injected back into the patient. This study is used to assess regional and global wall motion, ventricular function and cardiac chamber size but not myocardial perfusion.

Endocrine imaging

- **99mTc-pertechnetate:** For thyroid function. Patient is imaged within 15-30 minutes after injection.
- **99mTc-sestamibi or tetrofosmin:** for parathyroid function. Patient scanned at 20 minutes and 2 hours after injection.
- **Iodine-131 MIBG:** For neuroendocrine imaging. Thyroid blockade administered 5 days before scan. Patient imaged 1-2 days after injection of I131-MIBG
- **99mTc-MDP (methylene diphosphonate):** For bone scan. Imaged 2-5 hours after injection. Can be performed as SPECT.

Renal imaging

- **Tc99m-DTPA and Tc99m-MAG3:** For GFR estimation. Dynamic images acquired for 25-30 minutes after injection. Can give diuretics.
- **Tc99m-DMSA:** For cortical function e.g. scarring. Patient imaged 3 hours after injection. Static study, not functional.

CNS imaging

- **Brain SPECT with technetium-99m HMPOA:** Start imaging patient 20 minutes to 2-3 hours after injection.
- **Iodine 123 Ioflupane (aka DaTscan):** SPECT. Used in imaging Parkinson's disease. Thyroid blockade administered. Patient imaged 3-6 hours after injection.

Lung imaging

- **99mTc-DTPA aerosol:** For ventilation. Static image immediately after inhalation.
- **99mTc-MAA injection:** For perfusion. Imaged immediately after injection then static images taken from different angles.

Infection / inflammation imaging

- **Gallium-67 citrate:** Performed for regional or whole body imaging, planar or SPECT. Patient imaged at 48 hours and 72 hours.

Oncology imaging

- **Gallium 67 citrate:** For non-Hodgkin lymphoma, melanoma and hepatocellular carcinoma. Image on day 2 and 3.
- **99mTc-octreotide:** imaged at 2-4 hours and at 4 hours
- **18F-FDG PET:** Imaged at 30-60 minutes after injection for 5-60 minutes.

GI imaging

- **99mTc-mebrofenin:** For hepatobiliary function. Continuous dynamic imaging up to 60 minutes. Delayed imaging at 3-4 hours if needed.
- **Radiolabeled test meal using 99mTc-sulfur colloid:** For gastric emptying. Planar images taken 1 minute immediately after then repeated for 1 minute every hour.

2) Classification by radioisotope

Below is a summary of each radioisotope and the common uses. In the radioisotope header is the radioisotope, type of radiation emitted, method of production and half-life. For each radiopharmaceutical is the method of administration, whether it is used **in vivo** or **in vitro**, clinical use and whether it produces images or not. Despite the length of this table it is not exhaustive!

Carbon-11	**Positron**	**Cyclotron**	**20.3 m**	
C11-Choline	IV	In vivo	PET: suspected prostate recurrence	Imaging
C11-L-Methyl-methionine	IV	In vivo	Brain tumour imaging Parathyroid imaging	Imaging
Carbon-14	**Beta**	**Reactor**	**5730 y**	
C14-Glycocholic acid	Oral	In vitro	Breath test for small intestine bacterial overgrowth	Non-imaging
C14-Urea	Oral	In vitro	Breath test for H. pylori	Non-imaging
Chromium-51	**Gamma**	**Reactor**	**28 d**	
Cr51	IV	In vitro	RBC volume heart scan, RBC sequestration, GI blood loss	Non-imaging
Cr51-EDTA	IV	In vitro	GFR	Non-imaging
Cobalt-57	**Gamma**	**Cyclotron**	**279 d**	
Co57-Cyanocobalamin	Oral	In vitro	GI absorption	Non imaging
Fluorine-18	**Positron**	**Cyclotron**	**109 m**	
F18-FDG	IV	In vivo	Tumour imaging Myocardial imaging	Imaging
F18-Sodium fluoride	IV	In vivo	Bone imaging	Imaging
F18-Fluorocholine	IV	In vivo	Prostate cancer	Imaging
F18-Desmothoxyfallypride	IV	In vivo	Dopamine receptor imaging	Imaging
Gallium-67	**Gamma**	**Cyclotron**	**78.3 h**	

Ga67-Ga3+	IV	In vivo	Tumour imaging Infection / inflammation	Imaging
Ga67-Citrate	IV	In vivo	Hodgkin's disease, lymphoma, bronchogenic carcinoma Acute inflammation	Imaging
Gallium-68	**Positron**	**Generator**	**68 m**	
Ga68-Dotatoc	IV	In vivo	Neuroendocrine tumour	Imaging
Ga68-PSMA	IV	In vivo	Prostate cancer	Imaging
Indium-111	**Gamma**	**Cyclotron**	**1.81 d**	
In111-DTPA	Intraperitoneal	In vivo	Ventriculoperitoneal shunt patency	Imaging
In111-DTPA	Intra-cisternal	In vivo	Cisternography	Imaging
In111-leucocytes	IV	In vivo	Infection / inflammation	Imaging
In111-platelets	IV	In vivo	Thrombus imaging	Imaging
In111-Pentetreotide or Octreotide	IV	In vivo	Neuroendocrine tumour	Imaging
Iodine-123	**Gamma**	**Cyclotron**	**13.2 h**	
I123-Iodide	IV or oral	In vivo	Thyroid function Thyroid cancer metastases	Imaging
I123-MIBG	IV	In vivo	Neuroectodermal tumour imaging	Imaging
I123-ioflupane aka DaTscan	IV	In vivo	SPECT: Parkinson's disease	Imaging
Iodine-131	**Gamma and beta**	**Reactor**	**8.06 d**	
I131-Iodide	Oral	In vivo	Hyperthyroidism / thyroid cancer treatment	Therapeutic
I131-Iodide	IV or oral	In vivo	Thyroid metastases	Imaging
I131-MIBG	IV	In vivo	Neuroectodermal tumour imaging	Imaging
Krypton-81m	**Gamma**	**Cyclotron**	**13 s**	
K81m-gas	Inhalation	In vivo	Lung ventilation imaging	Imaging
Kr81m-aqueous solution	IV	In vivo	Lung perfusion imaging	Imaging
Oxygen-15	**Positron**	**Cyclotron**	**2.04 s**	

O15-water	IV bolus	In vivo	Cerebral blood flow Myocardial blood flow	Imaging
Strontium-89	**Beta**	**Reactor**	**50.5 d**	
Sr89-Chloride	IV	In vivo	Bone metastases treatment	Therapeutic
Technetium-99m	**Gamma**	**Generator**	**6.02 h**	
Tc99m-Pertechnetate	IV	In vivo	Thyroid uptake and imaging Stomach and salivary glands Meckel's diverticulum Brain imaging	Imaging
Tc99m-human albumin	IV	In vivo	Cardiac blood pool / peripheral vascular imaging Lung perfusion imaging	Imaging
Tc99m-Phosphonates and phosphates	IV	In vivo	Bone imaging Myocardial imaging	Imaging
Tc99m-DTPA	IV	In vivo	Renal imaging Brain imaging	Imaging
Tc99m-DTPA	Inhalation	In vivo	Lung ventilation	Imaging
Tc99m-DMSA	IV	In vivo	Tumour imaging Renal function	Imaging
Tc99m-Colloid	IV	In vivo	Bone marrow GI bleeding	Imaging
Tc99m-Colloid	Interstitial	In vivo	Lymph node drainage	Imaging
Tc99m-Colloid	Oral	In vivo	Oesophageal transit and reflux Gastric emptying	Imaging
Tc99m-HIDA	IV	In vivo	Functional biliary system	Imaging
Tc99m-denatured RBCs	IV	In vivo	RBC volume Spleen imaging	Imaging
Tc99m-whole RBCs	IV	In vivo	GI bleeding Cardiac blood pool	Imaging
Tc99m-MAG3	IV	In vivo	Renal imaging	Imaging
Tc99m-HMPOA	IV	In vivo	Cerebral blood flow	Imaging
Tc99m-examatazime labelled leucocytes	IV	In vivo	Infection / inflammation	Imaging

Tc99m-Sestamibi	IV	In vivo	Parathyroid / thyroid Myocardial	Imaging
Tc99m-Tetrosfosmin	IV	In vivo	Parathyroid Myocardial	Imaging
Tc99m-Tilmanocept	Interstitial		Lymphatic mapping with handheld gamma counter	Non-imaging
Thallium-201	**Gamma**	**Cyclotron**	**73.5 h**	
Tl201-Tl+	IV	In vivo	Thyroid tumour / parathyroid adenoma Myocardial	Imaging
Xenon-133	**Gamma**	**Reactor**	**2.26 d**	
Xe133-gas	Inhalation	In vivo	Lung ventilation	Imaging
Xe133 in isotonic sodium chloride solution	IV	In vivo	Cerebral blood flow	Imaging

6.5 Gamma Camera

The gamma camera is the equipment used to detect the distribution of radiopharmaceutical within the patient

Components:
- Collimator
- Radiation detector
  - Scintillation crystal
  - Photomultiplier tubes
- Electronics
  - Preamplifier

Collimator

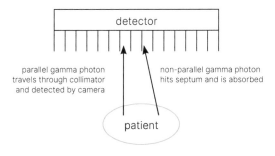

Figure 193 Collimator

When radiation is released from the patient it can exit at any angle and hit the detector in a location that doesn't correlate with the location of its origin. To overcome this, a collimator is used in which only gamma photons that travel parellel to the collimator will be accepted. Those travelling at an angle will hit the septum (usually lead), be absorbed and, therefore, not contribute to the image.

N.B. The collimator acts as a lens to reject photons that have a path that means they do not hit the camera in a location that corresponds to their original location i.e. its purpose is for spatial mapping. **It does not reject scatter.**

Features of the collimator

Hole direction

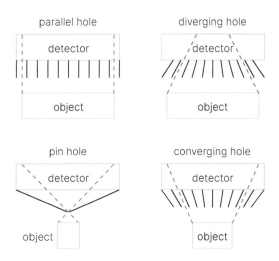

Figure 194 Types of collimator

- Parallel hole - these are the most common.
- Diverging hole - for a minified image
- Converging hole - for magnifying the image
- Pinhole - single-hole collimator for magnifying images of small objects e.g. thyroid

Hole formation

The holes can be created by:

- Crimped lead foil sheets (cheap but the gaps in the septae degrade image contrast)
- Drilling into a lead block (these give better image contrast as there are no gaps in the septae, but are more expensive)
- Casting from molten lead.

Septal thickness

The higher the energy of the emitted gamma photons the thicker the septae need to be to ensure maximum absorption of photons that hit them at an angle and, therefore, better rejection of non-perpendicular photons. Parallel hole collimators are classified as low, medium or high energy according to their septal thickness.

Classification	Photon energy (keV)	Septal thickness (mm)	Radionuclide
Low energy	150	0.3	99mTc
Medium energy	300	1	Indium-111
High energy	400	2	131I

Detector

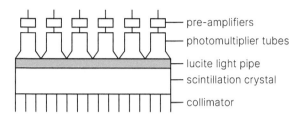

Figure 195 Gamma camera head

1) Scintillation crystal

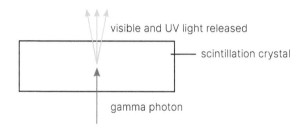

Figure 196 Scintillation

- The crystal is fluorescent i.e. when a gamma photon interacts it releases light photons (mixture of visible and UV light)
- Single crystal of sodium iodide with a small amount of thallium (NaI(Tl)). The thallium improves the light output.
- 6-13 mm thick
- Hermetically sealed in aluminium can

2) Perspex slab (light pipe)

- This sits between the scintillation crystal and the photomultiplier tubes
- Silicone grease is used to ensure good contact between the scintillation crys-

tal, the light pipe and the photomultiplier tubes.

3) Photomultiplier tubes (PMT)

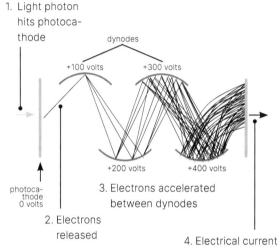

1. Light photon hits photocathode

dynodes

+100 volts   +300 volts

photocathode 0 volts

+200 volts   +400 volts

3. Electrons accelerated between dynodes

2. Electrons released

4. Electrical current collected at the anode (last dynode) which generates the current pulse that creates the signal

5. Signal received by pre-amplifier

Figure 197 Photomultiplier

- 30-100 PMTs sit behind the scintillation crystal
- The purpose of these is to multiply the small amount of light detected from the scintillation crystal to a large signal.

1. The light photons hit a photocathode at the entrance to the PMT.
2. The photocathode releases electrons in proportion to the amount of light that hits

it.

3. The electrons are attracted to the electrodes (dynodes) which have an increasingly positive charge along the PMT. This accelerates the electrons. As they accelerate, they gain kinetic energy resulting in multiple electrons being released from the dynode for each electron that hits it. This serves to multiply the original signal.
4. The total electrons hit the final anode and the current produced forms the signal received by the pre-amplifier.

4) Pre-amplifier

This converts the current produced at the anode of the PMT to a voltage pulse. The amplitude of the voltage pulse is directly proportional to the charge produced at the anode and, therefore, the amount of light received by the PMT, which is proportional to the number of gamma photons that hit the scintillation crystal.

Image Formation

1) Energy calculation

For each scintillation formed, the calculated absorbed energy (Z value) that caused it depends on the energy of the gamma photon that was emitted from the patient and the proportion of the energy that was absorbed into the crystal.

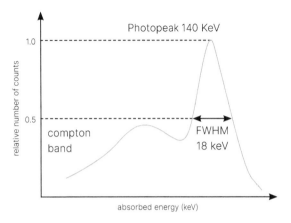

Figure 198 Range of energy absorbed by crystal

The gamma photon energy absorbed by the scintillation crystal depends on its interaction with that photon which results in a spectrum of Z values.

1. All energy absorbed: gamma photon interacts with crystal via photoelectric effect
2. Part of the energy absorbed: photon undergoes one or more Compton interactions

The spectrum has a peak (**photopeak**) that corresponds to the maximum gamma photon energy (for 99mTc this is 140 keV). The **Compton band** corresponds to photons that have undergone Compton interactions and, therefore, have a lower absorbed energy.

The photopeak should be very narrow but a variety of factors means that it often isn't. The width of the photopeak is measured as the **full width at half maximum (FWHM)**. This value is used to calculate the energy resolution of the crystal, which is given as a percentage:

Energy resolution = FWHM (keV) / photopeak energy (keV) x 100

2) Scatter rejection

If a gamma photon scatters within the patient's body (via Compton scatter) it will change direction and, therefore, will not hit the detector at a location corresponding to its location of origin. It is important to reject these scattered photons as they degrade the image contrast and spatial resolution. This cannot be done by the collimator and is, therefore, done electronically by a process called **energy discrimination**.

A gamma photon that scatters within the patient will never hit the scintillator with the full energy (i.e. it won't lie within the peak). Therefore, only gamma photons in the peak can be confidently identified as non-scattered radiation from the patient.

Usually a **20% acceptance window** is used centred on the photopeak. The acceptance window can be adjusted and more than one window can be used for radionuclides that have more than one photopeak (e.g. indium-111 has peaks at 172 and 247 keV). This is made possible by the Z values being displayed with a **multi-channel analyser** that allows more than one window to be set.

Key Point: Compton Band

Gamma photon energies within the Compton band can be due to:
- Unscattered photons that have undergone Compton interactions with the crystal
- Scattered photons that have undergone Compton interactions within the patient

Unfortunately these are indistinguishable and so energy discrimination will remove both the lower energy unscattered and scattered signals.

3) Image formation

Each PMT corresponds to a coordinate on the scintillation crystal. This is then mapped out onto a matrix. Each time a gamma photon that falls within the acceptable energy window is detected it is mapped on to its corresponding coordinate within the image.

Image acquisition is controlled by the user and may be terminated when:
- Preset number of counts obtained
- Preset time passed

4) Image display

The digital image is displayed upon a monitor with each pixel corresponding to a memory location in the matrix and the brightness / colour scale corresponding to the count number in that location.

Display can be manipulated and optimised by:
- Smoothing to reduce noise
- Windowing to increase contrast
- Interpolation increases the display matrix relative to the acquisition matrix which spreads the counts and makes the pixels less apparent
- Adding and subtracting images to extract quantified information

Summary

1) Collimator

- Series of holes separated by lead septae
- Rejects non-parallel gamma photons that do not hit the gamma camera in a location corresponding to their location in the patient
- Does not remove scatter

Hole direction
- Parallel: most common
- Diverging: to minify image
- Converging: for magnify image

- Pinhole: single-hole for magnifying small objects e.g. thyroid and tear ducts

Hole formation
- Crimped lead foil sheets: cheap but gaps in septae degrade the image
- Drilled lead block: no septal gaps so better image contrast but more expensive
- Casting from molten lead

Septal thickness
- Low energy: max keV 150, septae 0.3 mm, for 99mTc
- Medium energy: max keV 300, septae 1 mm, for Indium-111
- High energy: max keV 400, septae 2 mm, for 131I

2) Detector

Scintillation crystal
- Single crystal of sodium iodide with thallium. 6-13 mm thick
- Gamma photon hits - releases light photons (visible and UV light)

Light pipe
- With silicone grease ensures good contact between scintillation crystal and PMTs and spreads light across several PMTs

Photomultiplier tubes (PMT)
- 30-100 PMTs
- Multiply signal

1. Light photon hits photocathode
2. Releases electrons
3. Electrons accelerated between dynodes of increasingly positive charge. Multiple electrons released per electron that hits the dynode
4. Electrons hit final anode. Current produced forms signal that pre-amplifier receives

Pre-amplifier
- Converts current from anode into voltage pulse

3) Image formation

Energy calculation
- Gamma photon interactions with crystal:
  - Photoelectric - full energy absorbed by crystal
  - Compton - proportion of energy absorbed by crystal
- Calculated absorbed energy (Z value) spectrum with photopeak at maximum radioisotope energy
  - Energy resolution = FWHM

Scatter rejection
- Gamma photons that undergo Compton scatter in patient have lower energy
- Scatter electronically rejected via energy discrimination. Acceptance window around photopeak rejects gamma photons that have undergone Compton scatter

- Also reject gamma photons that are not scatter from patient but have undergone Compton scatter in crystal
- More than one acceptance window can be set

6.6   Planar Imaging

Types of Planar Imaging

Planar imaging is the acquisition of 2D nuclear images, similar to plain films in x-ray imaging.

1) Static

- Used for studies in which the distribution of the radiopharmaceutical is effectively static throughout the acquisition e.g. bone scan
- Inject → wait → image
- The time from injection to imaging depends on the study being performed.
- The total time of imaging can be determined by a preset time or a preset number of counts
- A static image can provide information on:
  - Organ size, shape and position
  - Regions of increased or decreased uptake
- **Examples**: DMSA renal scan, bone scan, lung perfusion scan

2) Dynamic

- Used for studies in which the distribution of the radiopharmaceutical changes rapidly with time
- Inject → image immediately → acquire series of frames over time
- The time between frames varies depending on the study being performed
- A dynamic study provides information on variation of radiopharmaceutical distribution over time
- **Examples**: MAG3 renal scan, gallbladder emptying scan, gastric emptying scan

3) Gated

- Used to study organs with regular physiological motion
- **Example**: cardiac gated blood pool imaging - acquisition is triggered by the R wave of the ECG. Images are then acquired. When the R wave occurs again the new images are overlaid onto the images from the previous cardiac cycle.

Image Acquisition

The operator can alter several variables during image acquisition depending on the nature of the scan being performed.

1) Collimator

The appropriate collimator needs to be selected for the study (more detail in **6.5 - Gam-**

ma camera section).

1. Low, medium or high energy collimator depending up the radionuclide used
2. General purpose, high resolution or high sensitivity collimator
   - High resolution gives better spatial resolution at the expense of a lower count rate and, therefore, longer imaging times. Usually used when spatial resolution of small structures important e.g. bone scan
   - High sensitivity gives better count rates but lower spatial resolution. Usually used in dynamic imaging when count rate is more important than anatomy e.g. renography.
3. Parallel, diverging, converging or pinhole configuration

2) Number of counts

- The aim is to increase the count density to achieve a high signal to noise ratio (SNR). Count density is increased by:
  - Increasing imaging time
  - Increasing the amount of administered radiation
  - Ensuring acceptable gamma camera sensitivity

3) Matrix

- A larger matrix = more pixels in the image and, therefore, better spatial resolution.

But this comes at a cost of fewer counts per pixel (lower SNR) and higher processing power required.

- Small matrix = fewer, larger pixels but better SNR
- Typical matrices:
  - Static imaging: 256 × 256
  - Dynamic imaging: 128 × 128 or 256 × 256
  - Gated cardiac imaging: 64 × 64

4) Orientation

- The orientation of the images can be changed by altering the position of the patient or the camera
- Oblique / lateral imaging can help differentiate structures that are overlying each other on the AP views
- If an object larger than the field of view needs to be imaged (e.g. whole body bone scan) this can be done by:
  - Continuous: the couch travels between the camera heads at a constant speed and the computer reconstructs the image
  - Step and shoot: 4-6 static images are taken along the body and these are then stitched together during processing

5) Position of camera

- The gamma camera should be as close to the patient as possible to optimise spatial resolution and signal. A smaller air gap means the radioactivity has a smaller spread as it passes through the collimator and, therefore, better spatial resolution.

- A small air gap can be achieved with infrared autocontouring which maintains the camera at a close but safe distance from the patient as the gamma camera scans along.

6) List mode acquisition

- In dynamic and gated imaging we can record the time information with the detected radioactivity. We can then split the signal acquired according to different time intervals. However, this requires a large amount of computer memory to be able to store all the data including data that will not be incorporated into the final image.

Image Display

1) Lookup tables

- The relationship between the pixel signal count and the displayed colour / brightness is determined by a lookup table.
  - Linear = linear relationship between signal count and displayed value.
  - Non-linear (i.e. logarithmic or exponential) = used for images in which the signal is concentrated in an area that is not of interest (e.g. the bladder in a bone scan) to prevent the majority of display values being used to display this small number of pixels and reduce overall contrast.

2) Contrast enhancement

The display of pixel brightness / colour is adjusted by adjusting the windowing. The displayed values should be set so that the pixels of interest are displayed best.

Image Processing

1) Image filtering

Convolution is used to smooth and sharpen the image by altering the count density values in the image (i.e. not just adjusting the display of the counts).

2) Region of interest (ROI)

A region of interest analysis can be used to calculate the total number of counts in a specified area. The region can be drawn by the user or drawn automatically by the processing system. If counts are calculated for anterior and posterior views the mean can be taken which corrects for depth (e.g. in a DMSA)

3) Time activity curves

The count rate in a specific ROI on a study can be shown over time in the form of a graph. This can then be used to calculate parameters and display these as a colour / brightness scale rather than just the number of counts:

- Time to reach the peak
- Area under the curve
- Washout rate of a radiopharmaceutical

Summary

1) Types of imaging

- Static: inject → wait → image
- Dynamic: inject → image immediately → acquire series of frames over time
- Gated: inject → image and collect timing data → reconstruct data into time periods

2) Image acquisition

- Collimator:
  - Low, medium or high energy
  - General purpose, high resolution or high sensitivity
  - Parallel, diverging, converging or pin-hole
- Count number:
  - Increase imaging time
  - Increase administered radiation
- Matrix size:
  - Large matrix = better spatial resolution but more noise
- Orientation of camera / patient:
  - Oblique / lateral for superimposed structures
  - Continuous or step-and-shoot for large object
- Position of camera:
  - Close as possible to patient - use infrared contouring system.

3) Image display

- Lookup tables: linear or non-linear
- Contrast enhancement: i.e. windowing

4) Image processing

- Image filtering with convolution
- ROI analysis
- Time activity curves in dynamic / gated studies

6.7 SPECT Imaging

Single photon emission computed tomography (SPECT) is the method of obtaining cross-sectional nuclear images (similar to CT in x-ray imaging).

- Single photon:
  - SPECT uses single gamma photon detection that are produced by gamma photon decay
  - c.f. PET which uses the simultaneous detection of the two gamma photons that arise from positron decay
- Emission:
  - Radioactivity used to create image is emitted from patient rather than transmitted through patient from an outside source as is done in x-ray imaging
- Computed tomography:
  - Slices are imaged that can be reconstructed into 3D data

SPECT can be used to image any radiopharmaceutical in which:

- The distribution does not change significantly during the image acquisition time (20-40 minutes)
- Acquisition time long enough for sufficient amount of gamma photons to be collected

Equipment

1) Camera / detector

a. Single head gamma camera
- Rotated around the patient during image acquisition
- Long image acquisition times
- No longer commonly used

b. Multiple head gamma camera
- Dual head, large field of view camera
- Housed on a gantry with slip ring technology that can rotate the cameras around the patient
- The cameras can be positioned in either an H-configuration or an L-configuration relative to each other

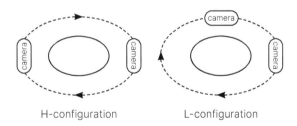

Figure 199 Camera head configuration

2) Hybrid SPECT/CT

- X-ray source and x-ray detector array placed between the gamma camera heads

- Anatomical CT and functional SPECT images then fused
- CT information can also be used to correct for attenuation in the SPECT images

3) Gantry

Needs to have:
- Accurately aligned centre of rotation
- Constant rotational speed
- Detectors aligned parallel to axis of rotation

4) Collimator

Important to use high resolution collimator
- Maximise spatial resolution throughout depth of the patient
- Reduce image distortion during reconstruction

Hole direction
- Parallel holes
  - Hole and septae size as uniform as possible
- Non-parallel holes
  - Can only be used with circular (i.e. not body contouring) orbits e.g. heads

Collimator type
- Fan beam collimator
  - Used for brain imaging
  - Utilises magnification - uses more of the detector field of view to collect the image data

Ensure smallest camera-patient distance but maintain safe distance
- Infra-red beams fitted to collimator face that enable automatic body contouring to minimise the detector-patient distance and optimise image quality
- Fitted with pressure sensitive safety devices to prevent any contact between the collimators and the patient

5) Patient table

- Needs to be comfortable due to long image acquisition times
- Low attenuation of gamma photons to allow photons to pass through and enable 360 degree acquisition

Image Acquisition

1) Matrix

- Determines maximum resolution and image noise (counts per pixel)
- Modern dual headed system = 128 × 128 matrix
- To reduce image noise (at expense of resolution):
  - Increase slice thickness
  - Smoother reconstruction filters
  - Display slice data in 64 × 64 pixel matrix

2) Views

- 20-40 sec per projection frame
- Heads rotated in continuous or 'step and shoot' mode

3) Minimising artefacts

- Minimise patient movement
- Injection site (very high count density) should be kept out of the field of view
- Arms above heads for chest and abdominal imaging to remove radiation attenuation and minimise patient-detector distance

4) Specific scans

- Cardiac SPECT
    - Heart is located off centre
    - Imaged over 180 degrees from LPO to RAO projection with heads in L mode to reduce detector distance and attenuation in tissues
    - ECG gating used to demonstrate cardiac wall motion (8 frames per cardiac cycle acquired into 64 × 64 matrix for each projection angle)

Reconstruction

objects being imaged

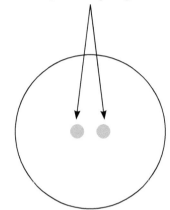

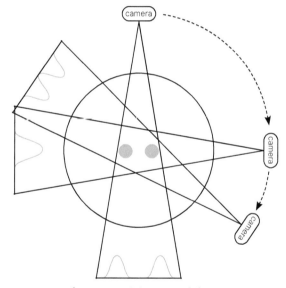

1. camera rotates around the objects taking 1D images

Figure 200 Back projection 1

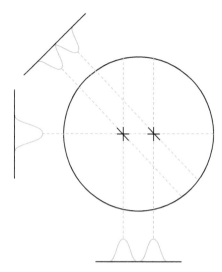

2. A new slice image is created from the acquired data using "backprojection". This image is very noisy. The objects are just visible as "stars" at the points at which the backprojections intersect.

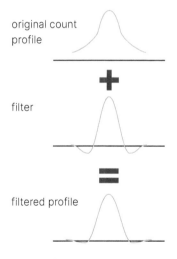

original count profile

filter

filtered profile

3. To reduce the star artefact the profiles are filtered prior to carrying out backprojection (filtered backprojection). This serves to smooth the calculated image.

Figure 201 Back projection 2

1. Creation of 1D profiles from each projection angle

- As the camera rotates around, it creates a 1 dimensional view of the measured radioactivity for each angle.

2. Filtering of profiles

- Compromise between noise reduction (degree of smoothing) and preservation of image (resolution)
- Smoothing usually defined by cut-off or critical frequency of the filter (maximum spatial frequency present in image)

3. Processing of data to create reconstructed slice image

- Back projection or iterative reconstruction of the filtered profiles create the reconstructed slice image. More detailed accounts of backprojection and iterative reconstruction is available in 3.3 - Acquiring an Image (Part 2).

Correcting for attenuation:

- Analytical method: apply algorithm that assumes uniform attenuation and then adjusts pixel counts depending on distance from camera and edge of patient
- Direct measurement: CT data can be used to calculate an attenuation map and adjust the pixel counts according to this

6.8   PET Imaging

Similar to SPECT, PET is a form of tomographic nuclear imaging. However, PET relies on the near simultaneous detection of the pair of gamma photons that are released from an annihilation of a positron and an electron.

Annihilation

1. Positron decay

In positron decay a positron (represented as e⁺, β⁺ or e) is released, which is the antiparticle of the electron (e⁻). A positron has the same mass and magnitude of charge except that the charge is positive.

$$^A_Z \text{Parent} \longrightarrow {^A_{Z-1}} \text{Daughter} + e + ve$$

Figure 202 Positron emission

Radionuclides that decay via positron emission typically have a larger proportion of protons compared to the number of neutrons (see 1.1 - Atomic Structure). These proton-rich radionuclides are typically produced in a cyclotron.

The energy difference between the parent and daughter nuclei must exceed 1.022 MeV (2 × 0.511 MeV) for positron decay to occur.

2. Positron travels through matter

1. As it travels it collides with atoms losing energy and causing ionisation (main method of radiation dose deposition in patient)
2. As it collides the positron is deflected and the path becomes tortuous. The length of the path depends upon the number of collisions and the starting energy of the positron. This means that the distance between where the positron is emitted and where it annihilates is variable.

3. Annihilation

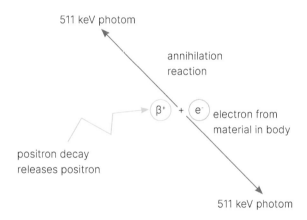

Figure 203 Annihilation

3. Shortly after its production a positron will **annihilate** with an electron
4. The energy from annihilation is released in the form of two photons with an energy of 511 keV
5. If the electron and positron are at rest before annihilation (initial momentum is zero) after annihilation the momentum of the

photons must remain zero. To achieve this the annihilation photons must travel in opposite directions (final momentum is zero)

1) PET radiopharmaceuticals

The most commonly used radionuclide is fluorine-18 and the most common pharmaceutical label is fluorodeoxyglucose (FDG). FDG is a tracer for glucose metabolism

PET Scanner

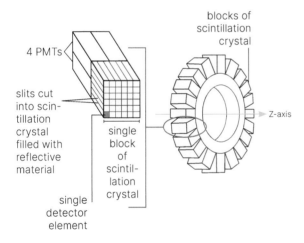

Figure 204 PET scanner

Blocks of scintillation crystals (detector blocks) are arranged in a circle mounted on a gantry in one or two rows. The ideal qualities of the scintillation crystal are:

- High linear attenuation coefficient (LAC) for the 511 keV photons
- High ratio of photoelectric to Compton interactions

- High number of light photons produced per gamma photon absorbed
- Short scintillation light decay time

1) Scintillation crystal

- The NAI scintillation crystal used in SPECT and planar imaging not suitable for PET as LAC not enough for the annihilation photons which have a higher energy of 511 keV
- Most commonly used scintillator in PET imaging is bismuth germanate (BGO)
- But the light output and light decay time are inferior to NaI
- Newer materials, such as lutetium oxyorthosilicate (LSO and gadolinium oxyorthosillicate (GSO) are being developed which have more suitable properties
- Each scintillation detector block viewed by four photomultiplier tubes (see 6.5 - Gamma Camera section for more information on PMTs)
- Block of crystal subdivided by cutting smaller blocks into the scintillation crystal ("called detector elements") and placing a reflective material in the slits to prevent cross-talk of the light photons between the elements

Forming an Image

As annihilation produces two gamma photons that travel in opposite directions, this is used to determine which photons should be used to form the image. Two opposite detector elements must simultaneously detect a gamma photon (to within 1 nanosecond) for those photons to contribute to the image. The simultaneous gamma photon by opposite detector elements is called a **coincidence** and the line between the two detector elements is called the **line of response**. The detector elements also encode the total energy deposited by the gamma photons.

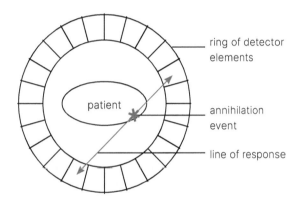

Figure 205 Line of response

N.B. this is how collimation is achieved in PET. The lead collimator grids that are used in planar imaging and SPECT are not required.

1) Data acquisition

2D vs 3D acquisition

In **2D acquisition** only coincidences confined to a single slice of the patient are used to form the image. This is achieved by using a collimator ring made of tungsten (which is highly attenuating) to reject photons that reach the detec-

tor at an angle and, therefore, are likely to have originated in a different slice of the patient.

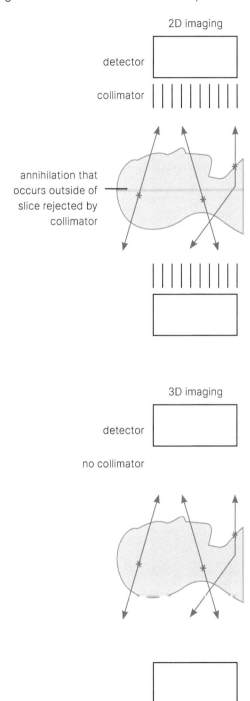

Figure 206 2D and 3D imaging

In **3D acquisition** no collimator is used and coincidences from a much greater volume of tissue are accepted. This method enables a higher total count rate due to more coincidences by allowed to reach the detector. It is useful when there is relatively little scatter / administered radiation such as in brain or paediatric imaging.

Unwanted coincidence rejection

Unwanted coincidences cause artefactual lines of response to be calculated which do not correspond to the true location of the annihilations.

- Increased **scatter** coincidence occurs when:
  - More material to travel through (e.g. body vs brain imaging)
  - 3D acquisition
  - Solution: Energy discrimination (see 6.5 - Gamma Camera section for more information). However, the photopeak window is wide due to poor energy resolution of the scintillators so scatter coincidence not eliminated
- Increased **random** coincidence occurs when:
  - 3D acquisition
  - Increased administered radioactivity
  - Increased duration of coincidence window

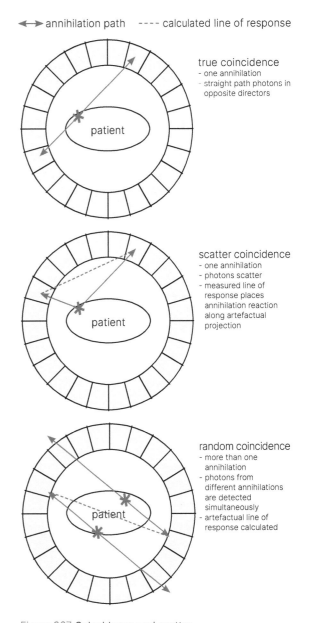

annihilation path   calculated line of response

true coincidence
- one annihilation
- straight path photons in opposite directors

scatter coincidence
- one annihilation
- photons scatter
- measured line of response places annihilation reaction along artefactual projection

random coincidence
- more than one annihilation
- photons from different annihilations are detected simultaneously
- artefactual line of response calculated

Figure 207 Coincidence and scatter

Attenuation correction

Problem:
- Attenuation is greater in PET than in SPECT due to the longer path the photon must travel through the patient.

Correction:
1. **Assume** cross-sectional shape and uniform LAC of tissue at 511 keV
2. **Measure** the transmission of 511 keV photons through the patient for each line of response. A radioactive rod source (gallium-68) that gives rise to annihilation radiation is rotated around inside the detector gantry without the patient and then with the patient. This allows a calculation to be made correcting for the attenuation by the patient.

Normalisation

Problem:
- Individual detector elements differ in dimensions and fraction of scintillation light photons that reach the PMTs. Same radiation source may not produce same response in every detector element.

Solution:
- Rotating rod source used without object in the scanner to calculate the correction factor required for differences in the individual detector elements
- Correction factor = measured counts for line of response / average counts for all lines

Dead time

Problem:
- Following the detection of a photon a detector element cannot detect another photon for a period of time (dead time)
- Results in loss of counts especially in 3D scanning

Solution:
- Dead time measured and mathematical algorithms that take into account detector behaviour applied to extrapolate from measured counts

Radioactive decay

Problem:
- Radioactivity decays as the scanner moves down the patient. The longer the delay from start to finish the more the radioactivity will have decayed

Solution:
- Counts corrected for radioactive decay

2D acquisitions are reconstructed using filtered back projection or iterative reconstruction (see 3.3 - Acquiring an Image (Part 2))

.

Summary

1) Annihilation

- Decay of radionuclide by positron decay
- Positron released → travels through body → interacts with electron (annihilation) → release two gamma photons of 511 keV that travel in opposite directions

2) PET scanner

- Gadolinium oxyorthoscillicate scintillation blocks arranged in circle around gantry
- Each block connected to 4 PMTs
- Blocks sectioned into detector elements with reflective material between them

3) Forming an image

- Coincident gamma photons (detected by two detectors along line of response within 1 nanosecond of each other) only are recorded and contribute to image

Data acquisition

- Dimensions
  - 2D uses collimator to accept only photons from a given slice
  - 3D doesn't use collimator, images larger volume of tissue
- Unwanted coincidence rejection
  - Scatter coincidence from photons created in same annihilation
  - Random coincidence from photons created in different annihilations

Data correction

- Attenuation correction
  - Assume cross-section shape and uniform LAC of tissue or
  - Use radioactive rod source (gallium-68) with and without patient to calculate correction required
- Normalisation
  - Rod source calculates correction factor for individual detector elements (i.e. differences between different lines of response)
- Dead time
  - Time following detection in which detector insensitive to further incident gamma photons calculated and counts corrected for
- Radioactive decay
  - Correction made for radioactive decay as scanner travels down the patient

Data reconstruction

- Uses filtered back projection or iterative reconstruction

6.9　NM Image Quality

As with other modalities the three major factors that determine image quality are:

- Contrast
- Noise
- Spatial resolution

Contrast

In radionuclide imaging contrast is created by the differential uptake of a radiopharmaceutical agent. Lesions can have negative (smaller lesion activity than surrounding tissue) or positive (larger lesion activity) contrast.

1) Subject contrast

The subject contrast is a property of the imaged object i.e. the radioactivity level in a lesion relative to healthy tissue. It is calculated as:

$$C_S = (A_L - A_T) / A_T$$

Where:
C_S = subject contrast
A_L = activity per unit volume of the lesion
A_T = activity per unit mass of the healthy tissue

2) Image contrast

Image contrast is the difference in the display between the lesion and surrounding healthy tissue. It is represented as the counts per unit area and also called the **count density** or information density. It can be expressed as counts per pixel.

$$C_I = (S_L - S_T) / S_T$$

Where:
C_I = image contrast
S_L = counts per unit area of the lesion
S_T = counts per unit area of the health tissue

3) Factors reducing image contrast

- **Smaller** subject contrast
- Greater **background gamma radiation** (for positive contrast radiopharmaceuticals)
  - Background radiation gives a count density that is overlayed on to the whole image.
  - Sources of background radiation include radioactivity in tissue above and below the lesion and other radioactive sources (in vicinity of patient or in environment)
- Using a **collimator**: photons penetrate septae and count density decreases

- **Scattered** radiation from patient
- **Attenuation** of the gamma radiation from a deep lesion which is much greater than for surrounding healthy tissue
- Greater patient **movement**
- Low spatial resolution of the **gamma camera**

Noise

Radionuclide imaging is an inherently noisy investigation. Too much noise will impair detectability of an object, especially if it is a low contrast object.

Structured noise:
- Non-random count density that interferes with object of interest due to:
  - Uptake in structure that is not of interest e.g. muscle uptake in PET after exercise, bowel uptake of gallium-67 citrate
  - Imaging system artefacts e.g. non-uniformity of the gamma camera

Random noise:
- Aka statistical noise or quantum mottle
- Due to random variations in count density as a result of random activity of radioactive decay
- More significant contributor of noise

1) Calculating noise

Relative noise (noise contrast) decreases as the count number (signal) increases.

$$\sigma = \sqrt{N}$$
$$\downarrow$$
$$SNR = N/\sigma = N/\sqrt{N} = \sqrt{N}$$
$$\downarrow$$
$$C_N = \sigma/N = \sqrt{N}/N = 1/\sqrt{N}$$
$$\downarrow$$
$$C_N = 1/\sqrt{AS}$$

Where:
σ = random noise (a standard deviation)
N = counts
SNR = signal to noise
C_N = noise contrast
A = area
S = count density

2) Factors reducing noise

- Longer acquisition **time**
- Increased **activity** of radiopharmaceutical (for given acquisition time)
- More sensitive **gamma camera** (however, increasing the sensitivity to decrease the relative noise also decreases the spatial resolution and contrast)

Spatial Resolution

Spatial resolution is quantified as the full width at half maximum (FWHM) measurement on a graph of counts or count rates vs distance. This is either measured when a radioactive point source (point source function, PSF) or when a line source (line source function, LSF) is imaged. The LSF is more commonly used. A Fourier transform of the LSF gives the modulation transfer function (MTF) which quantifies how accurately the image represents the object.

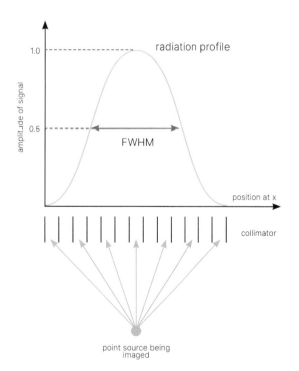

Figure 208 Point source function

1) Intrinsic spatial resolution (R_I)

The intrinsic spatial resolution is the maximum resolution achievable by the detector and electronics and depends upon many factors:

- Energy and linearity correction of scintillation
- Range of light in scintillation crystal. A thicker crystal means more spread and variation in the depth of the signal which reduces spatial resolution
- Higher gamma photon energy = more scintillation photons = smaller statistical variation which improves spatial resolution
- Optimised collection and detection of scintillation photons: good optical coupling and photomultiplier tube (PMT) shape (square or hexagonal better than circular), more PMTs
- Only PMTs above certain voltage contribute to signal (eliminates noise)

Intrinsic spatial resolution at 140 keV is between 2.5 mm FWHM (0.4 lp/mm) and 4 mm FWHM (0.25 lp/mm).

2) Collimator spatial resolution (R_c)

For a parallel hole collimator the collimator spatial resolution is:

$$R_C \approx d(1 + b/h)$$

Where:

R_c = collimator spatial resolution

d = hole diameter

b = distance from radiation source to collimator

h = hole length

From this equation you can see that resolution is improved by using a collimator with long holes of small diameter positioned as close to the patient as possible. However, there is still rapid degradation of spatial resolution the deeper the imaged object lies. Taking images from different orientations helps to minimise this.

3) System spatial resolution (R_S)

The R_S takes into account the intrinsic and the collimator spatial resolution to give the spatial resolution of the whole system.

$$R_S = \sqrt{(R_I^2 + R_C^2)}$$

Where:

R_S = system spatial resolution
R_I = intrinsic spatial resolution
R_C = collimator spatial resolution

4) Factors reducing resolution

- Low intrinsic spatial resolution of the **gamma camera**
  - Thick scintillation crystal
  - Small number of PMTs
  - Low threshold for PMT voltage to contribute to signal
- Low spatial resolution of the **collimator**
  - Large diameter holes
    - Short holes
    - Far from patient
- Increased patient **motion**
- Imaging deeper structures
- Large display **pixels**
- Increased **scattered** radiation
  - Improved with narrower energy acceptance window

PET image quality

Contrast

- Tomographic technique overcomes reduced contrast caused by radiation in front of and behind the lesion
- Random and scatter coincidences reduce contrast

Noise

Noise reduced by increasing sensitivity of the system which is determined by:

- Intrinsic detector efficiency
  - Scintillation crystal with higher LAC and more depth = better absorption of gamma photons = greater sensitivity
- Geometric detection efficiency
  - Higher number of gamma photons that reach detector = greater sensitivity
  - Better in 3D than 2D acquisition
- Width of photopeak acceptance window
  - Wider photopeak acceptance window = greater sensitivity
  - However, also increases scatter coin-

cidence detection rate which reduces contrast

Resolution

- Positron range
  - Distance from site of disintegration to annihilation
  - Longer range = poorer spatial resolution
  - ^{15}O is 2 mm, ^{18}F is better at 0.6 mm
- Non-colinearity of the annihilation photons
  - If positron or electron have residual momentum at time of annihilation the angle between the paths of the two gamma photons produced will not be exactly 180°
  - The greater the deviation the poorer the spatial resolution
- Detector element size
  - Smaller elements = better spatial resolution
- Thickness of crystal
  - Thicker crystal = poorer resolution
  - Resolution better through centre than periphery of detector ring
- Reconstruction filter
  - PET has much higher count rate sensitivity than SPECT and so noise is less of a problem
  - PET images can be reconstructed with much higher spatial frequency

Summary

1) Nuclear imaging

Contrast

- Subject contrast = property of imaged object
- Image contrast = property of the displayed image
- Reduced by:
  - Small subject contrast
  - High background radiation
  - Collimator
  - Scatter
  - Deep lesions being more attenuated
  - Patient movement
  - Low gamma camera spatial resolution

Noise

- Structured: non-random due to uptake in structures not of interest or imaging system artefacts
- Random
- Reduced by:
  - Long acquisition time
  - Increased radiopharmaceutical activity
  - More sensitive gamma camera

Spatial resolution

- Measured as full width at half maximum (FWHM)
- Intrinsic spatial resolution: maximum resolution achievable by detector and electronics
- Collimator spatial resolution: improved by

using collimator with long holes of small diameter positioned as close to the patient as possible

- System spatial resolution: takes into account intrinsic and collimator spatial resolution
- Reduced by:
  - Low intrinsic spatial resolution of gamma camera
  - Low spatial resolution of collimator
  - Patient movement
  - Deeper structures
  - Large display pixels
  - Increased scatter

2) PET

Contrast
- Tomographic technique overcomes reduced contrast from overlying structures
- Noise
- Reduced by increased sensitivity of system:
  - Higher intrinsic detector efficiency
  - Higher geometric detection efficiency
  - Wider photopeak acceptance window

Resolution
- Reduced by:
  - Longer positron distance from disintegration to annihilation
  - Non-colinear annihilation photons
  - Larger detector elements
  - Thicker crystals
  - Different reconstruction filter

6.10 NM Artefacts

- Injection site will cause high radiotracer activity
- Extravasation of injection causes uptake in lymph nodes

- Malfunction of gamma camera system
  - Photomultiplier tube (PMT) failure
  - Cracked or broken scintillation crystal
  - Correction matrix failure
  - Cracked crystal
  - Differences in detector sensitivity

- Attenuation can be caused by:
  - Objects worn by the patient e.g. belt buckles
  - Breast attenuation especially breast prosthesis
  - Diaphragmatic attenuation: especially in patients that are obese, have ascites, on dialysis
- Patient motion causes misalignment of reconstructed images
- Urinary contamination

- Head and neck
  - Brain cortex
  - Waldeyer's ring
  - Salivary glands
  - Extra-ocular muscles
  - Larynx in excessive talking
- Muscles
  - Stress-induced tension - trapezius and paraspinal muscles
  - Hyperventilation - diaphragm
  - Insulin - skeletal muscle
  - Vigorous exercise
- GIT / GUT
  - Caecum / right colon more glucose avid
  - Renal collecting system, ureters and bladder
  - Uterine uptake in menstruation
- Miscellaneous
  - Lactating breasts
  - Myocardial uptake post-prandially
  - Brown fat
  - Thymus in children

- Centre-of-rotation error
  - In SPECT, if presumed centre-of-rotation doesn't match actual axis of rotation back-projection will be affected

- Misregistration between radionuclide and CT images
- All CT related artefacts
- Truncation
  - SPECT field of view is larger than CT field of view
  - No CT data available for attenuation correction of the SPECT images

6.11 NM Quality Assurance

There is a legal requirement for quality assurance (QA) for all equipment used for medical exposure as specified in Ionising Radiations Regulations 2017 (IRR17).

Gamma Camera

Intrinsic measurement = when collimator removed

System measurement = with collimator

1) Uniformity

When irradiated by a uniform source the gamma camera should produce an image in which all pixels have the same count value. **The uniformity depends on the spatial linearity and energy response of the system.**
- Daily figures for uniformity acquired
- + 2SD from mean = remedial actions required

Intrinsic uniformity
- When collimator is removed
- Measured using point source of Cobalt-57
- Measured with point source positioned on central axis at 5x the diameter of the crystal (reduces variations in photon flux that reach detector to < 1%)

System uniformity:
- When collimator in place
- Measured using flood source. Either liquid filled with technetium-99 or plastic resin with Cobalt-57
- Acquired with linearity, energy and sensitivity corrections applied

2) Spatial resolution

Qualitative measurements
1. Anger pie phantom: segments with holes of different diameters separated by a distance of 4x the hole diameter
2. Quadrant bar phantom: four sets of lead bars of different spacing

Quantitative measurements
- Image a point or line source and calculate the full width at half maximum (FWHM)
    - Rayleigh criterion = FWHM is minimum separation required between two line sources to be seen as separate
- Emission phantom (e.g. Williams' liver phantom) - thinned phantom (hot spots) or perspex discs of different thicknesses (cold spots) layered over a radioactive source to assess resolution with different depths

3) Linearity

- Measures spatial distortion of an image
- Parallel line equal spacing phantom (PLES) imaged

4) Sensitivity

- Measures proportion of emitted radiation that is detected within the photopeak of the collimated gamma camera
- Image small phantom containing known amount of radioactivity measured for a known amount of time at a distance of 10 cm from the camera face

5) Count rate capability

- Measures ability of gamma camera to record count rate linearly as the count rate increases
- Usually expressed as 20% count rate loss - the count rate at which the recorded value is 20% lower than the expected value
- The lower recorded value is usually due to dead time

6) Energy resolution

- Spread of the recorded energy of incident gamma photons
- Measured as the FWHM of the photopeak

(maximum energy recorded energy of incident gamma photons)
- Energy resolution = FWHM / energy photopeak x 100%

SPECT

1) Centre of rotation

- Reconstruction assumes centre of rotation matches centre of detector gantry
- Measured by point source of technetium-99m in centre of field of view but offset by ~15cm from axis of rotation

2) Overall performance

- Measured using Jaszczak phantom - a cylindrical, liquid filled filled with rods and spheres

7

Radiation is present in the environment naturally and we are all exposed to some extent. The effect this radiation has on humans depends on the type, source and level of radiation and on the age of the patient. Legislation guides dose limits for staff and public and the dose reference levels (DRLs) for patients undergoing medical exposure. DRLs give an idea of the doses for standard-sized patients, but the dose may be larger for larger patients. Strictly, there are no dose limits for patients but the key guiding principle for patient, staff and public doses is ALARP (As Low As Reasonably Practicable).

This chapter covers the sources of radiation to staff, how the dose received is measured and how to protect against radiation exposure.

7.1	Effects of Radiation	259
7.2	Legislation	264
7.3	Radiation Protection	270
7.4	Dosimetry Badges	273
7.5	Patient Dosimetry	275

7.1   Effects of Radiation

Ionising Radiation

Ionising radiation is electromagnetic (EM) radiation that causes ionisation of atoms. The minimum energy needed to ionise any atom is approximately 10 eV.

Ionising radiation includes:
- X-rays
- Neutrons
- Beta particles
- Alpha particles

When the radiation interacts with the body damage is caused to **irradiated** cells by two mechanisms:
- **Indirectly**: ionisation produces free radicals which then damage DNA and cell membranes
- **Directly**: release of energy from ionisation event is enough to break molecular bonds directly

It also damages **non-irradiated** cells via:
- **Genomic instability in progeny** of cells: DNA defects passed on
- **Bystander effect**: release of chemicals and transmitters affect cells around the irradiated cell

Dividing cells are most sensitive to radiation when in **G2 and mitosis**. The more rapidly a cell is dividing, the greater its sensitivity

Sources of radiation
- Terrestrial
- Radon - accounts for about 50% of the average annual dose to people in the UK (some of course will get more, some zero). Emits alpha particles
- Radionuclides in food - especially potassium-40 (half-life of billions of years)
- Cosmic rays

Background radiation
Average effective dose in the UK is **2.7 mSv/year***
- 2.3 mSv from natural sources (0.006 mSv/day)
- 0.4 mSv from medical exposures

Dose at which there is a statistically significant increase in risk of cancer = 100-200 mSv

*Source: Ionising radiation: dose comparisons (published 18 March 2011 by Public Health England)

Measuring Radiation Dose

Name	Definition / formula	Pros and cons	Units
Absorbed dose	Energy deposited per unit mass of tissue	Doesn't take into account effect for different types of radiation or sensitivity of different organs irradiated	Gray (Gy) (1 Gray = 1 joule/kg)
Equivalent dose	Absorbed dose to tissue x radiation weighting factor	Takes into account effectiveness of different radiation types in producing biological damage	Sievert (Sv)
Effective dose	Sum of (equivalent dose x tissue weighting factor)	Sensitivity of different tissues to radiation taken into account	Sievert (Sv)

1) Equivalent dose

Equivalent Dose = Absorbed dose to tissue x radiation weighting factor
(summed for all types of radiation)

Different types of ionising radiation deposit different amounts of energy. This is measured by their **Linear Energy Transfer (LET)** or the density of energy deposition along the track of a photon or particle.

Low LET: x-rays, gamma rays, beta-particles. These are of high energy but pass through material quickly and deeply which leaves less time for energy to be deposited in any one area along its track.

High LET: alpha particles, neutrons. These are heavy and don't travel as far so all their energy is deposited into a small area.

This is then used to calculate the **Radiation Weighting Factor (W_R)**, the higher the W_R the more energy is deposited and the higher the equivalent dose from that type of radiation.

Radiation	Radiation weighting factor (WR)
X-ray and gamma ray (photons)	1
Beta particles and positrons	1
Protons	2
Alpha particles, fission fragments, heavy ions	20
Neutrons	A continuous function of neutron energy (see ICRP103 for graph/formula)

For x-rays, gamma rays and beta particles the W_R is 1 and so the equivalent dose in Sieverts is numerically the same as the mean absorbed dose in gray.

2) Effective dose

Effective dose = sum of (Equivalent dose x tissue weighting factor)

Each tissue in the body has a different sensitivity to radiation - its **Tissue Weighting Factor**. The Effective Dose takes this into account. The higher the tissue weighting factor, the higher that tissue's sensitivity to radiation i.e. the gonads have a higher sensitivity to radiation than skin. The below table shows the tissue weighting factors as stated in ICRP (2007).

Organ	Tissue weighting factor
Skin, bone, brain, salivary glands	0.01
Bladder, oesophagus, liver, thyroid	0.04
Gonads	0.08
Red bone marrow, colon, lung, stomach, breast, remainder of tissues	0.12

Effects of Radiation

The effects of radiation are down to how much and where the energy is deposited. A large weighting factor (W_R) leads to highly localised damage whereas gamma/x-rays deposit energy/dose over a much greater range. Thus, ingestion of alpha emitters (e.g. Radon) can have a large effect on the sensitive lining of the lung for instance.

1) Deterministic vs stochastic effects

Effects are either deterministic or stochastic.

Deterministic	Stochastic
Appear above a given threshold	No threshold to effects
The **severity** of the effect increases with dose	The **probability** of the effect increases with the dose
Effects occur within days of the exposure	Effects may happen years after exposure
Includes tissue effects e.g. erythema	Includes only cancer and genetic mutations

Risk of stochastic effects

The risk of stochastic effects is linked to the effective dose. For adults, the risk of inducing a cancer is approximately 5% per Sv. Therefore, for a 1 mSv effective dose (e.g. an abdominal x-ray), the risk is 1 in 20,000 of inducing a cancer. For comparison, the lifetime natural incidence of cancer is 1 in 2 or 1 in 3.

Children have a higher probability of radiation damage as they are developing and growing and there is more time for them latent effects of radiation to manifest in lateral life.

Deterministic effect thresholds

Exposed tissue	Net effect	Absorbed dose required for effect (Gy)	Time for effect to develop
	Initial erythema	2	2-24 hours
Skin	Erythema	3-6	1-4 weeks
	Hair-loss	3-4	2-3 weeks
Lens of eye	Cataract	3-5	Years
Bone marrow	Depression of blood formation	0.5	3-7 days
Gonads	Temporary sterility in males	0.15	3-9 weeks
	Permanent sterility	3.5-6	3 weeks

2) Acute whole body exposure

Whole body absorbed dose (Gy)	Principle organ involved	Time between exposure and death (days)
1-6	Bone marrow	3-60
5-15	GIT and lungs	10-20
>15	CNS	1-5

3) Pregnancy

Radiation-related risks throughout pregnancy depend upon the stage of the pregnancy and the absorbed dose. The highest risk is during the early fetal period, then the 2nd trimester, and finally the 3rd trimester. Preconception irradiation of either parent's gonads has not been shown to result in a higher risk of cancer or malformations in their children.

To cause malformations, typically to the central nervous system, the threshold is ≥100-200 mGy. These levels are very rarely reached with CT or conventional x-ray scans but can be reached with fluoroscopically guided interventional procedures of the pelvis or radiotherapy.

In females of child-bearing age there must be an attempt to determine whether the patient is, or could be, pregnant before exposure to radiation. One missed menstruation in a regularly menstruating woman should be considered positive for pregnancy until proven otherwise.

The natural childhood risk of cancer is approximately 1 in 500. From the table below you can see that the risk of childhood cancer is very low for most studies. At the highest doses, however, the childhood cancer risk can be double the natural risk.

Examination	Typical fetal dose (mGy)	Risk of childhood cancer per examination
X-ray skull; teeth; chest; thoracic spine; breast CT head +/- neck ^{51}Cr GFR measurement ^{81m}Kr lung ventilation scan	0.001 - 0.1	<1 in 1,000,000
CTPA ^{99m}Tc lung ventilation scan	0.01 - 0.1	1 in 1,000,000 to 1 in 100,000
X-ray abdomen; pelvis; hip Barium enema CT pelvis, chest and liver ^{99m}Tc lung perfusion scan; thyroid scan; DTPA; MAG3; DMSA; white cell scan	0.1 - 1.0	1 in 100,000 to 1 in 10,000
X-ray lumbar spine Intravenous urography Barium enema CT lumbar spine; abdomen ^{99m}Tc bone scan; cardiac blood pool scan; myocardial scan; cerebral blood flow scan ^{18}F PET tumour scan	1.0 - 10	1 in 10,000 to 1 in 1,000
CT pelvis; pelvis and abdomen; pelvis, abdomen and chest ^{99m}Tc myocardial scan ^{18}F PET/CT whole body scan	10 - 50	1 in 1,000 to 1 in 200

4) Breastfeeding

Some radionuclides are excreted in breast milk. It is recommended to suspend breastfeeding in the following situations:

- Completely after ^{131}I therapy
- For 3 weeks after ^{131}I, ^{125}I, ^{67}Ga, ^{22}Na and ^{201}Tl
- For 12 hours after ^{131}I hippurate and all ^{99m}Tc compounds except the below
- For 4 hours after ^{99m}Tc red cells, DTPA and phosphonates

References

ICRP, 2000. Pregnancy and Medical Radiation. ICRP Publication 84. Ann. ICRP 30 (1)

Wall, B. F., Meara, J. R., Muirhead, C. R., Bury, R. F., & Murray, M. (2009). Protection of pregnant patients during diagnostic medical exposures to ionising radiation. London: Royal College of Radiologists

7.2   Legislation

The two main pieces of legislation are:
- **IR(ME)R 2017:** deals with exposure to patients for medical and non-medical procedures (also IR(ME)R 2018(NI) and IR(ME)R (amendment) 2018)
- **IRR 17:** deals with exposure to employees and the public

For Nuclear Imaging, there is specialised legislation:
- **EPR 16 (previously RSA 93):** deals with storage and disposal of radioactive substances. Governs institutions.
- **CDG 2009 (previously RM(RT)R 2001):** deals with transport of radioactive substances

The Ionising Radiation (Medical Exposure) Regulations (2017) (IRMER 2017)

Governs all medical exposures and, since 2017, non-medical exposures to patients.
- Justification (net risk to patient in when considering risk of radiation and risk of not having the investigation)
- Optimisation (lowest dose that gives an image quality sufficient for diagnosis to be made. This does not mean the best image quality achievable with the equipment)

- Clinical audit
- Training
- Research exposure
- Medico-legal exposure
- Significant accidental or unintended exposures (SAUE)
  - Need to minimise the possibilities of incidents occurring
  - Includes cases of operator, procedure or equipment failure

A new requirement in the updates is that patients must be informed of the benefits and risks prior to the exposure taking place. Comforters and carers must be exposed knowingly and willingly indicating they, too, must be consented and made fully aware of the potential risks of radiation exposure. Also, licensing of practitioners and employers/facilities for the administration of radioactive substances has now been brought into IRMER.

** The main mantra of IRMER is ALARP **

As Low As Reasonably Practicable

1) Diagnostic Reference Levels (DRLs)

National Diagnostic Reference Levels are available on the gov.uk website. This gives a guideline of doses, not legal limit (there is no limit for patients but doses should be as low as reasonably practicable). These will vary from centre-to-centre, patient-to-patient, and with the complexity of the case (e.g. fluoro/interventional). Doses are audited every three years and the median shouldn't vary significantly from the DRL. There are also local DRLs in each hospital/trust which are usually lower than the national DRLs. Examples of DRLs can be found in the Appendix.

2) Roles and responsibilities

Referrer
- Health care professional entitled in accordance with employer's and local procedures to request and refer individuals for medical exposure
- Required to supply practitioner with sufficient medical information

Practitioner
- Required to justify all medical exposures and decide if exposure is in patient's best interest (e.g. person who vets requests)
- Can be the radiologist or radiographer

Operator
- Carries out and optimises the medical exposure
- Includes radiographer (pressing the exposure button, identifying patient, processing images, checking pregnancy status, etc) and technician performing annual quality assurance tests
- May have responsibility for authorising

exposures under written guidance from a practitioner e.g. radiographers in walk in chest x-ray lists can justify AND carry out procedure, i.e. practitioner and operator
- Responsible for optimisation (ALARP)

Employer
- Implements IRMER and allocates individuals to roles
- Provide written procedures and protocols
- Ensure staff are appropriately trained
- Respond where an incident has occurred

Medical Physics Expert
- Requires national recognition certificate
- Involved in:
  - Patient dosimetry
  - Equipment management
  - Optimisation
  - Advice on regulatory compliance

3) Summary

- Referrer doesn't need to justify procedure
- Practioner justifies exposure
- Operator optimises exposure, ensures ALARP followed, and operates image intensifier in fluoroscopy (may also be practitioner)
- One person can perform many different IRMER roles. The person pressing the exposure button is an operator, even if they are also the practitioner. In some cases, such as dental exams, one person can be the referrer, practioner and operator.

Ionising Radiation Regulations 2017 (IRR17)

IRR17 can be found on the legislation.gov.uk website. These regulations were produced under the Health and Safety at Work Act 1974 and designed to minimise radiation exposure to **employees and members of the public**. They are enforced by the Health and Safety Executive (HSE) and outlined in the Approved Code of Practice and guidance.

- Designed to ensure exposure to workers and members of the public follows ALARP
- Final responsibility for radiation safety lies first and foremost with the employer. In an NHS Trust this is the CEO.

1) Roles and Responsibilities

Radiation protection advisor

- Usually an expert physicist and should be trained in the use of radiation and have thorough knowledge of the associated hazards and their control
- Must have a certificate of competence issued by a body recognised by the HSE
- Advises on:
    - Identification and designation of controlled and supervised areas
    - Calibration of monitoring equipment
    - Risk assessments
    - Drawing up of local rules and contingency plans
- Quality assurance programmes

Radiation protection supervisor

- Appointed by employer
- Ensures local rules are being complied with
- Must known what to do in an emergency
- Must always be present on site
- There can be more than one radiation protection supervisor for each controlled area

Employees

- Not knowingly expose themselves or others to ionising radiation to a degree that is greater than necessary
- Make full and proper use of Personal Protective Equipment and report any defects in it
- Inform the employer about suspected incidents

Radiation risk assessment

- This is mandatory before stating a new activity or changing an activity involving ionising radiation
- Identify hazards
- Decide who may be harmed and how
- Evaluate the risks and decide on precautions
- Record your findings and implement them
- Review your assessment and update if necessary
- The risk assessment informs the local rules

2) Dose limits per calender year

To limit stochastic effects the effective dose limits are:

Employees and trainees ≥18 years old	20 mSv or 100 mSv in any period of five consecutive calendar years subject to maximum equivalent dose of 50 mSv in any single calendar year	Dose limit to abdomen of person of reproductive capacity	13 mSv in any consecutive 3 months
Trainees <18 years old	6 mSv (i.e. < 3/10 of adult dose)	Any person (not carer or comforter) that may be exposed to ionising radiation resulting from medical exposure of another person	5 mSv in any period of 5 consecutive calendar years
Anyone <16 years old or any person other than employee or trainee	1 mSv	Dose to fetus of pregnant employees	1 mSv for remainder of pregnancy

To prevent deterministic effects the **equivalent dose limits** in a calendar year are:

Area	Employees and trainees 18 years old or more	Trainees under 18 years old	Any person (not carer or comforter) who may be exposed resulting from medical exposure of another person
Lens of the eye	20 mSv in a calendar year averaged over 5 years with no single year exceeding 50 mSv	15 mSv	15 mSv
Extremities	500 mSv	150 mSv	50 mSv
Skin	500 mSv	150 mSv	50 mSv

3) Classified workers

This is anyone who is likely to receive:

- Effective dose of >6 mSv in a year (3/10 of dose limit)
- Equivalent dose of greater than 3/10 of any dose limit i.e.
  - >15 mSv/yr to lens
  - >150 mSv/yr to skin or extremities

Classified workers must:

- Must have a medical examination before being designated
- Must have periodic review of health at least once a year
- Must be at least 18 years old
- Records of doses received by classified workers must be kept until the person has, or would have, reached 75 years old and at least 30 years from when the record was made

4) Designation of special areas

Controlled areas

- Any person working in the area is likely to receive an effective dose of >6 mSv, 15 mSv to the lens, or equivalent dose of >3/10 of any relevant dose limit
- External dose rate exceeds 7.5 mSv/h over a working day
- Dose rate less than 7.5 mSv/h when averaged over a working day BUT the instantaneous dose rate at any point exceeds 100 mSv/h
- Any person who enters or works in area must follow special procedures to restrict significant exposure

Supervised area

- Required if anyone working in the area is likely to receive a dose >1 mSv/yr or an equivalent dose of >1/10 of any relevant dose limit (i.e. more than the dose limits for the general public)

5) Reporting overexposure

In England, under IR(ME)R, any significant accidental or unintended exposures (SAUE) of patients should be reported to the Care Quality Commission (CQC). Where workers or members of the public are over-exposed with radiation the incidence is reported to the Health and Safety Executive (HSE) under IRR(17). The criteria for notification of patient doses are outlined in the following table (values for England only).

Accidental exposure

Exposure category	Criteria for notification
All modalities including therapy	≥3 mSv effective dose (adult)
	≥1 mSv effect dose (child)

Unintended exposure

Exposure category	Criteria for notification
Intended dose <0.3 mSv	≥3 mSv effective dose (adult)
	≥1 mSv effect dose (child)
Intended dose 0.3 mSv to 2.5 mSv	≥10x more than intended
Intended dose 2.5 mSv to 10 mSv	≥25 mSv
Intended dose >10 mSv	≥2.5x more than intended
Interventional / cardiology	Where there has been no procedural failure AND either: the dose is ≥10x the local DRL OR there are observable deterministic effects excluding transient erythem
Radiotherapy pre-treatment planning scans	If CT planning scan needs to be repeated twice to obtain appropriate data set (i.e. 3 scans in total including the intended scan)
Foetal - all modalities	Where there has been a failure in the procedure for making pregnancy enquiries AND the resultant foetal dose is 1 mGy or more
Breast feeding infant - nuclear medicine only	Where there has been a failure in procedure AND the resultant infant effective dose is ≥1 mSv

Source: https://www.cqc.org.uk/guidance-providers/ionising-radiation/irmer-incident-notification-codes-categories-criteria

Nuclear Medicine Department

IR(ME)R (MARS 78 now revoked)
- Regulates administration of a radioactive substance
- Do not apply to substances that are naturally radioactive or administered for properties other than their radioactivity
- Administration of Radioactive Substances (ARSAC) license granted to site or practitioner
    - Site license: whole scope of practice (diagnosis, therapy and research). Inidicative list of practioners.
    - Practitioner license: for justification. Option to include research.
- Certificates are valid for 5 years and, following amendments, for a further 5 years

Environmental Permitting Regulations 2016
- Governs storage and safe disposal of radioactive materials
- Imposes requirements for traceability, record-keeping and contamination monitoring and security of radioactive sources
- Regulated by the Environment Agency
- Registration certificates are awarded to the sites of work, not individuals

Carriage of dangerous goods and use of transportable pressure equipment 2009
- Govern the transport of radioactive substances by road

References

Britain, G., & Health and Safety Commission. (2018). Work with Ionising Radiation: Ionising Radiations Regulations 2017: Approved Code of Practice and Guidance. HSE books.

Desai, R., Brejza, P., & Cremona, J. (2004). The ionising radiation (medical exposure) regulations-IR (ME) R, Malta. World Journal of Nuclear Medicine, 3(suppl. 1), S107-S108.

7.3 Radiation Protection

Sources of Radiation

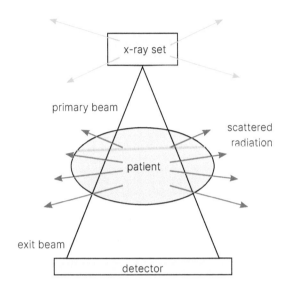

Figure 209 Sources of radiation exposure

1) Primary Radiation

Primary Beam: This refers to the x-ray beam prior to any interaction with the patient, grid, table or image intensifier.

Exit Beam: The beam that interacts with the detector is termed the exit beam and will have been significantly attenuated. However, the beam will have been heavily filtered and, consequently, will be harder and more penetrating than the primary beam.

2) Secondary Radiation

Leakage Radiation: This is leakage from the x-ray tube housing. However, this is limited to a maximum of 1 mGy/hr at 1 metre from the focus and, in practice, is usually much less. It doesn't contribute significantly to staff dose.

Scattered Radiation: This is a direct result of the Compton effect in the patient and **contributes the most to staff radiation dose**. The amount (fluence) of scatter depends on:
- Field size
- Volume of patient
- Quality of primary beam.

An increase in scatter can be caused by:
- Increased kV - number of photons proportional to square of applied potential
- Increased mA - number of photons directly proportional to tube current
- Increased energy
- Increased exposure time - no. photons directly proportional to length of time of exposure
- Larger volume exposed - more tissue for photons in x-ray beam to interact with. The tighter the collimation the less the scatter
- Position relative to patient - on the exit side of the patient the scatter is less as it has been attenuated by the patient as compared to scatter on the tube side (i.e. angular dependence, the greater the angle from the exit beam the greater the

scatter)

Minimising Staff Dose

1) Time

- Pulsed operation in fluoroscopy
- Last image hold in fluoroscopy enables decisions to be made without further exposure
- Virtual collimation

2) Distance

During acquisition phase, only essential personnel remain in the room and they are shielded. Radiation dose falls with distance as demonstrated by the **inverse square law**.

3) Shielding

Room design

Most rooms are designed so that any member of the public passing outside will not receive a dose from x-ray procedures being performed in that room of more than 0.3 mSv. Typical shielding for a busy x-ray room is 150 mm thick concrete walls or 2.0 mm lead ply strapped to an existing wall.

The operator's console/control room should provide areas behind which doses and dose rates are sufficiently low such that members of staff do not need to wear additional protective equipment. These include ceiling mounted, table mounted, intensifier mounted and mobile protective screens that are usually at lead equivalences of 0.5mm Pb.

Personal Protective Equipment

Local rules dictate what PPE is appropriate. These provide **no protection against primary radiation**. Lead gloves are often not recommended due to the risk of them getting in the primary beam, which would lead to the system increasing the exposure factors and giving a higher dose to both the patient and the staff.

Protection	Lead equivalence
Lead aprons	0.25 mm for 100 kV 0.35 mm for 150 kV
Thyroid shields	0.5 mm
Lead glasses	0.25 × 1.0 mm
Lead gloves	0.25 mm Modern gloves have 0.5 or 1.0 mm

Fluoroscopy and Interventional

1. **Overcouch configuration:** x-ray tube above the patient and beam directed downwards. This exposes the operator to more radiation as the scatter occurs upwards towards the upper body of the operator. These are used in C-arm systems but care must be taken to orient tube away from the operator during oblique

views.
2. **Undercouch configuration:** the intensifier is positioned above the patient as close as possible and, therefore, provides some shielding to the operator. The dose to staff is 10x less than in overcouch.

4) Pregnant/Breast Feeding Staff

When pregnancy is declared, a risk assessment should be carried out by the employer to make sure dose limits are adhered to. For declared pregnant staff the dose limit is 1 mSv to the fetus over the duration of the pregnancy which, generally, translates to a 2 mSv dose limit to the abdomen of the pregnant employee.

No extra precautions are necessary if breast feeding except if working in the nuclear medicine department.

7.4   Dosimetry Badges

There are three general groups of dosimetry badges:

1. Film badges
2. Thermoluminescent Detectors (TLDs)
3. Electronic Dosimeters

If an employee is provided with a dose badge they are required to wear them under IRR 17. They measure staff doses to ensure that dose limits are complied with and to deterine who should be classified.

Film Badges

These use a silver-halide film (similar to that used in plain film radiography). They are an old technology and have been largely replaced with TLDs.

Advantages
- Cheap
- Can distinguish between different energies of photons
- Can measure doses from different types of radiation
- Provide a permanent record
- Accurate for exposures > 100 millirem

Disadvantages
- Film fogging over time
- Prolonged exposures can adversely affect the film
- Not accurate to exposures < 20 millirem
- Must be developed and read by a processor, which is time consuming
- Must be changed every 1 month due to fogging over time

Thermoluminescent Detectors (TLDs)

This is the most commonly used dosimeter. To read absorbed radiation the TLD is heated and visible light is released from the crystal in proportion to absorbed radiation. This is then measured to calculate the amount of radiation the dosimeter has been exposed to. Calcium fluoride and lithium fluoride are commonly used. The TLD must be used in its casing as this applies filters to correct for deep and superficial absorption through the skin. Calibration post-read-out is still required to correct for differential absorption. The rate of changing the TLDs varies between institutions. Some institutions may use area monitoring instead of individual monitoring if the expected doses are low.

Advantages
- Can be made very small for finger/eye doses
- Can be reused

Disadvantages

- Cannot distinguish between different types of radiation
- More expensive than film badges
- Once read out, record is lost i.e. can't provide permanent record

Electronic Dosimeters

Most commonly used electronic dosimeter uses silicone diode detector. They can provide a direct electronic readout and live/real time readouts and don't need the processing that is required for the other types of dosimetry badges. Require yearly battery replacement and checking.

Advantages

- Very sensitive. Nearly 100x more sensitive than a TLD and can measure to nearest 1 µSv
- Good for measuring pregnancy doses

Disadvantages

- High initial cost

7.5 Patient Dosimetry

1) X-ray imaging

Factors that increase dose:
- Beam properties
  - Higher tube current (mA) and exposure time (s)
  - Wider collimation (reduces scatter and irradiated area)
  - Larger field of view (FOV)
  - Higher kVp (if we stick with the same mAs, more photons overall and more with higher energy. However, some higher energy photons pass straight through the patient)
- Scanner properties
  - No filtration
  - Use of a grid
  - Reduced receptor sensitivity
- Patient properties
  - Closer to focal spot (x-ray source)
  - Larger patient habitus (larger skin surface to absorb maximum dose)

2) Fluoroscopy

Factors that increase dose:
- Beam properties
  - Lower kVp (a less penetrating beam means more radiation absorbed, particularly on skin)
  - Continuous (vs pulsed)
  - Using a higher dose level setting
  - Larger area of collimation
  - Keeping x-ray tube over same anatomical area (maximum skin dose can be reduced by rotating and penetrating patient from different angles, called "dose spreading")
  - Whether fluoroscopy or acquisition mode is selected
- Scanner properties
  - Use of a grid
  - Increased electrical magnification (zoom modes)
  - Increased geometric magnification (i.e. moving patient closer to source)
  - Decreased distance between the tube and the detector/II
- Patient properties
  - Larger patient habitus (as for x-ray imaging)

3) CT imaging

Factors that increase dose:
- Beam properties
  - Higher tube current (mA)
  - Higher kV
  - Longer exposure time
  - Not using mA modulation
  - Wider collimation (however, if collimation too small system will compensate for reduced signal by increasing mAs / kVp)

- Scanner properties
  - Decreasing pitch (normally dose and pitch inversely proportional. However, some scanners automatically correct for pitch by maintaining same
  - Use of noise reduction algorithm allows lower dose to be used
- Patient properties
  - Smaller patient (more x-rays will penetrate to the centre and deposit a higher dose N B. a larger patient will receive more total x-rays but dose is measured per unit mass)

4) Nuclear imaging

Factors that increase dose:
- Increased amount of injected radioactivity
- Each radioisotope will deposit different doses
- Reduced drinking and urination results in slower loss of activity from the bladder, increasing patient dose

A.	Basic Science	278
B.	X-Ray Imaging	279
C.	CT Imaging	283
D.	Ultrasound Imaging	285
E.	MR imaging	286
F.	Molecular Imaging	288
G.	Radiation Dosimetry, Protection and Legislation	291
H.	Miscellaneous	295

A. Basic Science

1 atomic mass unit (amu) = 1/12 the mass of a carbon-12 atom

Maximum number of electrons in a shell = $2n^2$ (**n = shell number**)

Kinetic energy = $\frac{1}{2}mv^2$ (m = mass; v = velocity)

Frequency = 1 / T (T = time between successive peaks in seconds)

Velocity (c, ms^{-1}) = $f\lambda$ (f = frequency; λ = wavelength)

Intensity (E) = hf (h = Planck's constant; f = frequency)

Intensity (E) = h/λ

Intensity $\propto$ 1 / d^2 (d = distance)

	Relative mass	Charge	Symbol
Neutron	1	0	n
Proton	1	+1	p
Electron	0 (1/2000)	-1	e-

1 Becquerel (Bq) = 1 transformation per second

B. X-Ray Imaging

Heat (J) = kVe x mAs = w x kVp x mAs (kVe = effective kV, w = waveform, kVp = peak kV, mAs = current per second)

Temperature rise = energy applied / heat capacity

Compton scatter $\propto$ density / energy

Photoelectric LAC $\propto \rho Z^3 / E^3$ (ρ = density, Z = atomic number, E = energy)

Compton LAC = ρ / E

Factor of reduction = 2^{HVL} (HVL = half value layer)

Linear attenuation coefficient (LAC, cm^{-1}) = 0.693 / HVL

Mass attenuation coefficient (MAC, cm^2g^{-1}) = LAC / density

Image plate (IP) = barium fluorohalide activated with divalent europium ions. 0.3 mm

Red laser beam for read out
Light released in blue part of spectrum
Speed = 2000 / X (X = dose incident on IP)

Detective quantum efficiency (DQE) = SNR^2_{out} / SNR^2_{in} (SNR = signal to noise ratio)
- 0.25 for standard IP
- 0.12 for high resolution IP

Indirect DR

Scintillator layer = 500 μm layer of caesium iodide with thallium (CsI:Tl)
X-ray photon $\rightarrow$ ~3000 light photons in green spectrum
Matrix = amorphous silicon layer doped with hydrogen (a-Si:H)
Fill factor = sensitive area / overall area

Direct DR

Photoconductor = amorphous selenium (a-Se)

Maximum compression = 200 N (normal = 100-150 N)
Target/filter:
- General use: MoMo
- Dense breasts: MoRh or RhRh

Broad focal spot = 0.3 mm
Fine focal spot = 0.1 - 0.15 mm
Focus-to-film distance = 65-66 cm

Equipment

II window made of aluminium of titanium foil
Input phosphor:
- Sodium activated caesium iodide (CsI:Na)
- 400-500 μm thick,
- Produces light photons in blue spectrum

Photocathode:
- Antimony caesium (SbCs3)

Output screen:
- Silver-activated zinc cadmium sulphide (ZnCdS:Ag)
- 25-35 in diameter, few micrometres thick

Equations:

$G_{brightness} = G_{minification} \times G_{flux}$ ($G_{minification}$ = minification gain; G_{flux} = flux gain)

$G_{minification} = (D_{input} / D_{output})^2$ (D_{input} = diameter of input screen; D_{output} = diameter of output screen)

$G_x = L / X'$ (G_x = image intensifier conversion factor; L = luminance of the output; X' = entrance dose rate)

$G_{minification} \sim 100$

$G_{flux} \sim 100$

$G_x \sim 10\text{-}30$

Tungsten (W)
Characteristic radiation:
- Kα = 59.3 keV
- Kβ = 67.6 keV

Mass number (A) = 184

Atomic number (Z) = 74

Molybdenum (Mo)
Characteristic radiation:
- Kα = 17.5 keV
- Kβ = 19.6 keV

K-edge = 20 keV

Rhodium (Rh)

Characteristic radiation:
- Kα = 20.2 keV
- Kβ = 22.7 keV

K-edge = 23.3 keV

Subject contrast (c) $\propto (\mu_1 - \mu_2) \times t$ (μ = attenuation coefficient of object 1 and 2, t = object thickness)

Noise inversely proportional to √photons

Geometric unsharpness (U_g) = f x b / a (f = x-ray focal size; a = distance from x-ray source to front surface of object; b = distance from object to detector)

Magnification (M) = image size / object size = d2 / d1 (d2 = focal spot to detector; d1 = focal spot to object)

Sampling frequency = 2 x Nyquist frequency

8) Quality assurance

Required by IRR 1999. IPEM report 91 provides guidance.

Equipment tested	Frequency of testing	Method of testing	Performance criteria
X-ray tube output	1-2 months	Dose at various exposures measured with ionisation chamber at known distance	Repeatability: ■ Remedial = ± 10% ■ Suspension = ± 20% Consistency: ■ Remedial = ± 20% ■ Suspension = ± 50%
Light beam alignment	1-2 months	Light beam field compared to exposed field on film	Remedial = 1 cm misalignment on any side at 1 m from focal spot Suspension = 3 cm
Automatic exposure control (AEC) performance	1-3 months	Film exposed at different tube voltages and different perspex thicknesses to ensure consistent OD	Remedial = ± 0.3 OD relative to baseline Suspension = ± 0.5 OD relative to baseline
Low contrast sensitivity	4-6 months	Uses Leeds Test Object Ltd test object	Remedial = baseline ± 2 groups
DR/CR limiting spatial resolution	4-6 months	Uses lead grating resolution bar pattern	Remedial = baseline minus 25%
AEC ionisation chamber consistency	Annual	Expose ionisation chambers separately and compare (usually three)	Remedial = ± 0.3 OD relative to baseline Suspension = ± 0.5 OD relative to baseline

Equipment tested	Frequency of testing	Method of testing	Performance criteria
Focal spot	Annual	Pinhole: Pinhole radiographed and size, shape and inconsistencies of focal spot calculated from image produced Star test object: Radiating lead spokes radiographed and central blurred area size used to calculate focal spot size	
Filtration	Annual	Half value thickness / layer of filter determined and compared to available data to calculate filtration Should be equivalent to 2.5 mm aluminium	
Detector dose indicator repeatability and reproducibility	Annual		Remedial = baseline ± 10% Suspension = baseline ± 20%
Threshold contrast detail detectability	Annual	Test object with appropriate filter and kV imaged	
Uniformity of resolution	Annual	Fine wire mesh imaged	Remedial = increase in blurring from baseline
Scaling errors	Annual	Grid imaged with object of known length	Remedial = >2% deviation from object
Dark noise	Annual	No exposure or low exposure	Remedial = baseline + 50%
X-ray tube kV	1-2 years	Electronic kV meter measures kV at different exposure settings	Remedial = ±5% or ±5 kV from baseline Suspension = ± 10% or ± 5kV from baseline

C. CT Imaging

Detector array = 8 - 64 rows; 700 - 900 detectors per row

Single slice pitch = detector pitch = couch travel per rotation / detector width

Multislice pitch = beam pitch = couch travel per rotation / total width of simultaneously acquired slices

Hounsfield unit (HU) = CT number = 1000 x (ut - uw) / uw (ut = attenuation coefficient of tissue; uw = attenuation coefficient of water)
Focal spot: fine = 0.7 mm, broad = 1.0 mm)

Pixel size (d) = FOV / n (FOV = field of view; n = image matrix size)
Highest spatial frequency (fmax) = 1 / 2d

CT number values

Tissue	CT number (HU)
Bone	+1000
Liver	40 to 60
White matter	20 to 30
Grey matter	37 to 45
Intravascular blood	30 to 45
Fresh clotted blood	70 to 80
Muscle	10 to 40
Kidney	30
CSF	15
Water	0
Fat	-50 to -100
Air	-1000

Dose

Dose = mAs / pitch

Measurement	Definition	Equation	Unit
CT dose index (CTDI)	Dose to the detector from single gantry rotation		mGy
Weighted CTDI (CTDI$_w$)	Adjusted for spatial variation of dose	$\frac{1}{3}$ CTDI$_{centre}$ + $\frac{2}{3}$ CTDI$_{periphery}$	mGy
Volume CTDI (CTDI$_{vol}$)	Accounts for pitch	CTDI$_w$ / pitch	mGy
Dose length product (DLP)	Total dose along distance scanned	CTDI$_{vol}$ x distance scanned	mGy cm

Effective dose (E)	Physical effect of total radiation dose	1) Σ (H_T x W_T)
		2) E_{DLP} x DLP
		H_T = individual organ dose
		W_T = tissue weighting factor
		E_{DLP} = agreed value of E_{DLP} for whole region

D. Ultrasound Imaging

1) Equations

Audible range of soundwaves = 20 to 20,000 Hz

Medical ultrasound = 2 to 18 MHz

Speed of sound through tissue = 1540 ms

Velocity (c) = $\sqrt{k / \rho}$ (k = rigidity; ρ = density)

c = f λ (f = frequency; λ = wavelength)

Intensity (dB ratio) = $10 \log^{10} (I_1 / I_2)$ (I_1 = intensity 1; I_2 = intensity 2)

Acoustic impedance (Z, kg m^{-2} s^{-1}) = density x speed of sound in that material

Reflection coefficient (R) = $(Z_2 - Z_1)^2 / (Z_2 + Z_1)^2$

Beam weight = focal length x λ / D (λ = wavelength; D = diameter of PZT crystals)

2) Doppler

Resistive index (RI) = (peak systolic frequency - end diastolic frequency) ÷ peak systolic frequency

Pulsatility index (PI) = (peak systolic frequency - minimum frequency) ÷ time averaged maximum frequency

In low resistance artery: normal RI = 0.6 - 0.7; abnormal RI = 0.8 - 1.0

Nyquist limit = PRF / 2

3) Equipment

Piezoelectric material = ½ wavelength thick; 256 crystals

Matching layer = ¼ wavelength thick

Near field distance = $D^2 / 4\lambda$ (D = diameter of transducer; λ = wavelength)

Pulse repetition frequency (PRF) = frame rate x lines per frame

Distance of wave = time x velocity x 0.5

Depth of view = 0.5 x sound velocity / PRF

4) Safety

Thermal index (TI) = power emitted / that required to increase temperature by 1°c. Keep < 0.5

Mechanical index (MI) = peak negative pressure / $\sqrt{\text{ultrasound frequency}}$. Keep < 0.7. In fetal scanning <0.5

Time averaged intensity < 100 mWcm^{-2}

Total sound energy < 50 Jcm^{-2}

E. MR imaging

1) Equations

Larmor equation (F) = precessional frequency = K x B_0 (K = gyromagnetic ration; B_0 = strength of static magnetic field)

Larmor frequency of hydrogen at 1 Tesla = 42 MHz

Larmor frequency of hydrogen at 1.5 Tesla = 63 MHz

T1 = time for M_z (longitudinal magnetisation) to recover to 63%

T2 = time for M_{xy} (transverse magnetisation) to decay to 37%

Relaxation times at 1 Tesla

	T1 (ms)	T2 (ms)
Fat	250	80
Kidney	550	60
White matter	650	90
Grey matter	800	100
CSF	2000	150
Water	3000	3000
Bone, teeth	Very long	Very short

2) Sequence

Spin echo

- 90º RF → 180º RF rephasing pulse at TE/2 → Echo signal at time TE → repeat at TR
- Scan time = TR x no. GPE x NEX (GPE = phase encoding steps; NEX = number of signal aver-ages or slices)
- Turbo spin echo = TR x no. GPE x NEX / ETL (ETL = echo train length)
- T1 weighted: TR determines T1 signal. Short TR
- T2 weighted: TE determines T2 signal. Long TE
- Proton density: minimise T1 with long TR and minimise T2 with short TE

Inversion recovery

- STIR: short TI of 130 ms (TI = time to application of 180º inversion pulse)
- FLAIR: long TI of 2500 ms

Gradient recalled echo

- RF pulse of certain flip angle → gradient applied to rephase spins → echo signal at time TE → repeat at TR
- T1 weighted: large flip angle, short TE and short TR
- T2* weighted: small flip angle, long TE and short TR
- T2 weighted: can't achieve
- Proton density = small flip angle, short TE and short TR

MR Spectroscopy

1. Suppress water signal
   - CHESS
2. Select voxel / voxels
   - Single-voxel spectroscopy (SVS)
   - Multi-voxel chemical shift imaging
3. Acquire spectrum
   - PRESS and STEAM

	Metabolite	Frequency (ppm)	Role	Clinical relevance
ml	Myoinositol	3,6	Glial marker	>Raised in gliomas and MS Reduced in herpetic encephalitis
Cho	Choline	3,2	Cell membrane and metabolism marker	Raised in tumours and demyelination
Cr	Creatine	3,0	Energy metabolism marker	Constant peak
Glx	GABA, glutamine, glutamate	2,1 - 2,5	Intracellular neuronal transmitter	Raised in hepatic encephalopathy
NAA	N-Acetyl-Aspartate	2,0	Healthy neuronal marker	Raised in Canavan's disease Reduced in any condition resulting in loss of neurons
Lac	Lactate	1,3 doublet	Anaerobic respiration	Raised in ischaemia, seizures, tumours, mitochondrial disorders
Lip	Lipids	0,9 and 1,4		Raised in necrotic tumours
aa	Aminoacids	0,97		Raised in pyogenic abscesses

Localisation

1. Slice select along Z-axis with gradient
2. Segment along X-axis selected by frequency encoding
3. Segment along Y-axis selected by phase encoding
4. For 3D, segment along Z-axis selected by phase encoding
5. Wave decoded with Fourier transformation

K-space: periphery for fine detail, centre for contrast information

3) Angiography

Time of flight (TOF): non-contrast bright blood technique. Uses flow-related enhancement artefact

Phase contrast: non-contrast bright blood technique. Uses spin phase artefact.

Contrast enhanced: IV contrast bright blood technique

Contrast agents:

- T1 paramagnetic = shorten T1 = high T1 signal e.g. gadolinium, hepatobiliary agents that contain manganese
- T2 superparamagnetic = speeds up T2 decay = low T2 signal e.g. iron oxide based SPIOs and USPIOs

4) Artefacts

Local field inhomogeneity artefacts occur in frequency-encoding direction

External RF signal artefacts occur in phase-encoding direction

F. Molecular Imaging

1) Non-nuclear molecular imaging

- Contrast-enhanced ultrasound
    - Bubbles 1-4 µm
    - Filled with high-molecular weight gas e.g. perfuorocarbon and sulphur hexafluoride
    - Shell made typically of lipid
- Optical imaging
    - Bioluminescence: intracellular luciferase reacts with injected luciferin to produce detectable photon
    - Fluorescence: injected molecule activated with external light source and photon

emissions released from decay of excited state measured

- MR spectroscopy

2) Radiopharmaceuticals

- Cyclotron: Technetium-99m (molybdenum target), Fluorine-18 (Oxygen-18 target), Gallium-67, Thallium-201
- Nuclear reactor: Molybdenum (used to make Tc99m), Iodine-131, Xenon-133
- Radionuclide generator: Technetium-99m, Krypton-81

Radiopharmaceutical and clinical use	Method of decay	Method of production	Half-life
Carbon-11 C11-choline: prostate PET C11-L-Methyl-methionine: Brain and parathyroid	Positron	Cyclotron	20.3 m
Carbon-14 C14-Glycocholic acid: intestinal overgrowth C14-Urea: H. pylori	Beta	Reactor	5730 y
Chromium-51 Cr51: RBC Cr51-EDTA: GFR	Gamma	Reactor	28 d
Cobalt-57 Co57-Cyanocobalamin: GI absorption	Gamma	Cyclotron	279 d
Fluorine-18 F18-FDG: PET F18-sodium fluoride: bone F18-Fluorocholine: prostate F18-Desmothoxyfallypride: dopamine receptor	Positron	Cyclotron	109 m
Gallium-67 Ga67-Ga3+: tumour, infection, inflammation Ga67-Citrate: Hodgkins, inflammation	Gamma	Cyclotron	78.3

Radiopharmaceutical and clinical use	Method of decay	Method of production	Half-life
Gallium-68 Ga68-Dotatoc: neuroendocrine tumour Ga68-PSMA: prostate	Positron	Generator	68 m
Indium-111 In111-DTPA: VP shunt, cisternography In111-leucocytes: inflammation / infection In111-platelets: thrombus In111-Pentetreotide or Octreotide: neuroendocrine tumour	Gamma	Cyclotron	1.81 d
Iodine-123 I123-Iodide: thyroid function and mets I123-MIBG: neuroectodermal tumour I123-ioflupane aka DaTscan: Parkinsons	Gamma	Cyclotron	13.2 h
Iodine-131 I131-Iodide: hyperthyroid, thyroid cancer I131-MIBG: neuroectodermal tumour	Gamma and beta	Reactor	8.06 d
Krypton-81m K81m-gas: ventilation K81m-aqueous: lung perfusion	Gamma	Cyclotron	13 s
Oxygen-15 O15-water	Positron	Cyclotron	2.04 s
Strontium-89 Sr89-Chloride: bone mets	Beta	Reactor	50.5 d
Technetium-99m Tc99m-Pertechnetate: thyroid, stomach, Meckel's, brain Tc99m-human albumin: blood pool, lung perfusion Tc99m-Phosphonates: bone, myocardial Tc99m-DTPA: renal and brain Tc99m-DTPA: lung ventilation Tc99m-DMSA: tumour and renal Tc99m-Colloid: bone marrow, GI bleeding Tc99m-HIDA: biliary function Tc99m-denature RBCs: RBC volume, spleen Tc99m-whole RBCs: GI bleeding, cardiac blood pool Tc99m-MAG3: renal Tc99m-HMPOA: cerebral perfusion Tc99m-examatazime labelled leucocytes: infection / inflammation Tc99m-Sestamibi: myocardium, parathyroid Tc99m-TetrofosminL parathryoid, myocardium Tc99m-Tilmanocept: lymphatic mapping	Gamma	Generator	6.02 h
Thallium-201 TI201-TI: thyroid tumour, parathyroid, myocardium	Gamma	Cyclotron	73.5 h
Xenon-133 Xe133-gas: inhalation Xe133 in isotonic sodium chloride: cerebral perfusion	Gamma	Reactor	2.26 d

3) Equipment

Collimator:
- Low energy = 150 keV = 0.3 mm = ^{99m}Tc
- Medium energy = 300 keV = 1 mm = Indium-111
- High energy = 400 keV = 2 mm = ^{131}I

Scintillation crystal: sodium iodide with thallium (NaI(Tl)); 6-13 mm thick

System spatial resolution $(R_S) = \sqrt{(R_I^2 + R_C^2)}$ (R_I = intrinsic spatial resolution; R_C = collimator spatial resolution)

Energy resolution = FWHM (keV) / photopeak energy (keV) x 100 (FWHM = full width half maximum)

Scatter rejection = 20% acceptance window

4) PET imaging

Positron decay → annihilation with electron → two 511 keV photons
Scintillation crystal: bismuth germanate (BSO), lutetium oxyorthosilicate (LSO and gadolinium oxyorthosillicate (GSO)

5) Image quality

Subject contrast $(C_s) = (A_L - A_T) / A_T$ (A_L = activity per unit of lesion; A_T = activity per unit mass of healthy tissue)

Image contrast $(C_I) = (S_L - S_T) / S_T$ (S_L = counts per unit area of lesion; S_T = counts per unit area of healthy tissue)

Noise contrast $(C_N) = 1 / \sqrt{(AS)}$ (A = area; S = count density)

Collimator spatial resolution $(R_C) \approx d (1 + b/h)$ (d = hole diameter; b = distance from radiation source to collimator; h = hole length)

G. Radiation Dosimetry, Protection and Legislation

1) Dose

Absorbed dose (Gray) = energy deposited per unit mass of tissue

Effective dose (Sievert) = ∑(equivalent dose x tissue weighting factor)

Equivalent dose = ∑(absorbed dose to tissue x radiation weighting factor)

Background radiation = 2.7 mSv/year (2.3 mSv natural sources, 0.4 mSv medical exposure)

Radiation	Radiation weighting factor
X-ray and gamma ray	1
Beta particles and positrons	1
Neutrons < 10 keV	5
Neutrons 100 keV - 2 MeV	20
Alpha particles	20

External radiation: gamma and x-rays > beta > alpha

Internal radiation: alpha > beta > gamma and x-rays

2) Protection

Protection	Lead equivalence
Lead aprons	0.25 mm for 100 kV 0.35 mm for 150 kV
Thyroid shields	0.5 mm
Lead glasses	0.25 × 1.0 mm
Lead gloves	0.25 mm Modern gloves have 0.5 or 1.0 mm

Legislation

Ionising Radiation (Medical Exposure) Regulations (2017) (IR(ME)R 2017)
- ALARP - as low as reasonably practicable
- Governs all medical and non-medical exposures to patients

Ionising Radiation Regulations 2017 (IRR17)
- Under Health and Safety at Work Act 1974
- Minimises radiation exposure to employees and members of the public
- Enforced by Health and Safety Executive (HSE)

Effective dose limits per year:

Radiation workers > 18 years old	20 mSv 100 mSv in any 5 consecutive years, max dose of 50 mSv in any single year
Members of the public	1 mSv

Radiation workers < 18 years old	6 mSv i.e. 3/10 of adult dose
Dose limit to abdomen of person of reproductive capacity	13 mSv in any consecutive 3 months
Comforters and carers	5 mSv
Any other person / member of public (fetus counts as member of the public)	1 mSv
Pregnant employees dose to fetus	1 mSv for remainder of pregnancy

Equivalent dose limits per year:

Area	Employees and trainees >18 yo	Trainees <18 yo	Any other person
Lens of the eye	20 mSv	15 mSv	15 mSv
Extremities	500 mSv	150 mSv	50 mSv
Skin	500 mSv	150 mSv	50 mSv

Classified workers

Anyone who is likely to receive:

- Effective dose of > 6 mSv in a year (3/10 of dose limit)
- Equivalent dose of > 3/10 of any dose limit i.e.
    - > 15 mSv/year to lens
    - 150 mSv/year to skin or extremities

Controlled area

- Person likely to receive effective dose of > 6 mSv; 15 mSv to lens; or equivalent dose of > 3/10 of any relevant dose limit
- External dose rate exceeds 7.5 mSv/h over working day
- Dose rate < 7.5 mSv/h over working day BUT instantaneous dose rate at any point exceeds 100 mSv/h

Supervised area

Person working in area likely to receive dose of > 1 mSv/yr or equivalent dose of > 1/10 of any relevant dose limit.

Diagnostic reference levels

Source: www.gov.uk - National Diagnostic Reference Levels 19 August 2019

Radiograph	ESD per radiograph (mGy)	DAP per radiograph (Gy cm 2)
Abdomen AP	20 mSv	15 mSv
Chest AP	0.2	0.15
Chest PA	0.15	0.1
Cervical spine (AP and lat)		0.3
Knee (AP and lat)	0.6	0.6
Lumbar spine AP	5.7	1.5
Lumbar spine lat	10	2.5
Pelvis AP	4	2.2
Shoulder AP	0.5	
Skull AP/PA	1.8	
Skull lat	1.1	
Thoracic spine AP	3.5	1.0
Thoracic spine lat	7	1.5

Adult CT	CTDI vol per sequence (mGy)	DLP per complete examination (mGy cm)
ead	60	970
Cervical spine	21	440
Chest	12	610
High-resolution CT chest	4	140
Chest, abdomen and pelvis		1000
CT abdominal angiography	15	1040
CTPA	13	440
Abdomen	14	910
Abdomen and pelvis	15	745
Virtual colonoscopy	11	950
Kidneys, ureter and bladder	10	460
Urogram		170
Coronary CT angiography		170 - 380

Pediatric CT	CTD vol per sequence (mGy)	DLP per complete examination (mGy cm)
Paeds head: 0-1 y	25	350
Paeds head: >1-5 y	40	650
Paeds head: <5 y	60	860

Adult CT-PET / CT-SPECT	CTDI vol per sequence (mGy)	DLP per complete examination (mGy cm)
PET half body	4.3	400
SPECT bone scan	4.9	150
SPECT parathryoid	5.6	170
SPECT mIBG / octreotide	5.5	240
SPECT cardiac	21	36

Reporting overexposure:

Accidental exposure

Exposure category	Criteria for notification
All modalities including therapy	≥3 mSv effective dose (adult) ≥1 mSv effect dose (child)

Unintended exposure

Exposure category	Criteria for notification
Intended dose <0.3 mSv	≥3 mSv effective dose (adult) ≥1 mSv effect dose (child)
Intended dose 0.3 mSv to 2.5 mSv	≥10x more than intended
Intended dose 2.5 mSv to 10 mSv	≥25 mSv
Intended dose >10 mSv	≥2.5x more than intended
Interventional / cardiology	Where there has been no procedural failure AND either: the dose is ≥10x the local DRL OR there are observable deterministic effects excluding transient erythem
Radiotherapy pre-treatment planning scans	If CT planning scan needs to be repeated twice to obtain appropriate data set (i.e. 3 scans in total including the intended scan)

| Foetal - all modalities | Where there has been a failure in the procedure for making pregnancy enquiries AND the resultant foetal dose is 1 mGy or more |
| Breast feeding infant - nuclear medicine only | Where there has been a failure in procedure AND the resultant infant effective dose is ≥1 mSv |

Source: https://www.cqc.org.uk/guidance-providers/ionising-radiation/irmer-incident-notification-codes-categories-criteria

3) Nuclear medicine

MARS78: governs administration of radioactive substance

RSA93: governs storage and safe disposal of radioactive materials

Radioactive Material (Road Transport) (Great Britain) Regulation 2001: governs transport of radioactive substances by road

4) MRI safety

MHRA guideline for whole body exposure of **patients**

- Normal and pregnant 4 Tesla
- Controlled 8 Tesla
- Research no limit Tesla

MHRA guideline for exposure of **staff**

- < 2 T for whole body
- < 5 T for limbs
- < 0.2 T over 24 hours

Controlled area = 5 Gauss, 0.5 mT boundary

1 SAR = 1 W/kg = whole body temperature rise of 0.5°c

Operating mode	Rise of body core temperature (°c)	Localised temperature limits (°c)			SAR W/Kg
		Head	Trunk	Extremities	
Normal	0.5	38	39	40	2
Controlled	1	38	39	40	4
Restricted	2	39	40	41	> 4

Hearing protection needed at 90 dB

H. Miscellaneous

1) Resolution

Imaging modality	Resolution
Film screen radiograph	6 lp/mm
Digital radiograph	3 lp/mm
Film screen mammography	15 lp/mm
Digital mammography	5 to 10 lp/mm
Fluoroscopy	1 lp/mm
Direct subtraction angiography	2 lp/mm
Fluoroscopy - flat panel detector	3 lp/mm
CT: transaxial	2 lp/mm
CT: Z-sensitivity	2 to 0.4 lp/mm

2) Effective radiation dose

Procedure	Dose	Procedure>	Dose (mSv)
Abdominal			
CT Abdo/pelvis	10	XR lower GIT	3
CT colonography	6	XR upper GIT	6
Barium enema	7	XR pelvis	0.5
CNS			
CT head	2	XR cervical spine	0.2
CT spine	6	XR thoracic spine	1.0
CT neck	3	XR lumbar spine	1.5
		XR skull	< 0.1
Chest			
CT chest	7	XR chest	0.1

Procedure	Dose	Procedure>	Dose (mSv)
Cardiac CT	3	Mammography	0.4
Cardiac CTA	12 - 20		

Extremities

		XR hand / foot	0.005

Nuclear imaging

Brain PET (18F FDG)	14	DEXA	0.001
Brain perfusion (99mTc HMPAO)	9 to 10	Renal MAG3	2
Brain SPECT (99mTc sestamibi)	10	Renal DTPA	2
Bone scan	6	DaTscan brain	6 to 10
Heart stress (99mTc sestamibi)	9.4	V/Q	2.5
Thyroid scan	5	Gastric emptying	1
Whole PET/CT	24		

A

ABC (automatic brightness control) (in fluoroscopy) 70–71
ABPI measurement 130
absorbed dose 260, 260–276, 262, 292. See also dose, radiation
absorption, of sound waves 116
accelerating potential, in x-ray tube 21–22
acoustic enhancement, in ultrasound imaging 134
acoustic impedance (Z) 117
acoustic shadowing, in ultrasound imaging 134
active matrix, in digital radiography (DR) 38
actual focal spot 18. See also focusing, x-ray
AEC. See automatic exposure control (AEC) (in fluorography and radiography)
air gap
  in mammography 59, 61
  in nuclear medicine 234
  in x-ray imaging 44
aliasing
  in MR imaging 161–162, 199
  in ultrasound imaging 132
alpha particles 11
  decay model 12, 14
A-Mode (ultrasound) 119
amplification, and noise 48
angiography 72, 185–187
  Appendix notes 287
anode 17, 18–20. See also target (in x-ray tube)
  angles 18, 19
  Appendix notes 280
  cooling chart 20
  heating 19, 20
  heel effect 20, 59
  interactions and radiation 22–24
  tube rating 19
artefacts in MR imaging 161–162, 179–180, 186, 188, 196–201
artefacts in nuclear medicine 238, 239, 252–253
artefacts in ultrasound imaging 128, 132–133, 134–135
artefacts in x-ray imaging 37, 39–40, 50
  beam hardening. See beam hardening, x-ray
  correction/solutions 39–40, 72, 95, 104, 105, 105–106, 106–107, 108
  in CT imaging 103–109
  cupping artefact 104
  in digital subtraction angiography (DSA) 72
  measurement 108
  motion artefacts. See movement unsharpness/motion artefacts
  vignetting 72
atherosclerotic plaque removal 95
atomic mass unit (amu) 3
atomic number 3
  of target, and x-ray spectrum 26
  and x-ray attenuation 30, 31
atomic structure 3–5, 278
attenuation
  of gamma radiation 247
  of x-rays. See x-ray attenuation
attenuation correction
  in PET imaging 244
  in SPECT imaging 239
automatic brightness control (ABC) (in fluoroscopy) 70–71
automatic exposure control (AEC) (in fluorography and radiography) 54–55
  in mammography 60, 62
auto-ranging, in digital radiography (DR) 40

B

background radiation
  average effective dose 259
  and image contrast 246
backprojection, in CT imaging 91
bandwidth
  and chemical shift (in MR imaging) 162
  of RF pulse (in MR imaging) 158
  receiver bandwidth (in MR imaging) 162
beam alignment, x-ray 55
beam energy, x-ray 103
beam hardening, x-ray 32, 62, 95, 103
  cupping artefact 104
beam quality, x-ray 24
beam quantity, x-ray 24
beam steering, in ultrasound imaging 129
Becquerel (Bq) 11
beta particles 11
  beta minus decay model 12, 14
  beta plus decay (positron emission) model 12, 14
binding energy, of electrons 4
bioluminescence 213
bits and bytes 36
blood pool imaging 95

blurred edges 48–49
B-mode (ultrasound) 119, 119–120, 123
bone imaging
  nuclear medicine 232
breast feeding, and nuclear medicine 263, 272
breast imaging. See mammography
breast implant leakage 95
breast thickness and composition, and imaging 62
Bremsstrahlung radiation 23–24, 24–26
brightness gain, of image intensifier 65–66
British Medical Ultrasound Society (BMUS) 121
b-value, in diffusion weighted imaging 178

C

calibration
  gain calibration 39
  pixel-calibration 40
cancer, childhood, and fetal dose 262–263
cardiac gated blood pool imaging 232
cardiac imaging
  electron beam scanner 83
  nuclear medicine (NM) 219–220, 238
  ultrasound 128
Carriage of Dangerous Goods and Use of Transportable Pressure Equipment 2009 (CDG 2009) 269
cathode 17, 18. See also thermionic emission
  Appendix notes 280
cavitation risk, in ultrasound 121
CCD (charged coupled device) sensors, in fluoroscopy 70
central nervous system (CNS) imaging 220
characteristic radiation 22–23, 24, 24–26
chemical shift artefact, in MR imaging 162
classified workers (designated under IRR17) 267
coincidences, in PET imaging 243
collimation and collimator
  in CT imaging 80
  in gamma camera 225–226, 232–233, 237
  in SPECT imaging 237
  in PET imaging 242
  in planar imaging (nuclear medicine) 232–233
  spatial resolution 248–249, 249
comet tail artefact, in ultrasound imaging 135
compression, in mammography 61
Compton attenuation coefficient 28
Compton band 228, 229
Compton effect (Compton scatter) 27–28, 228
  vs photoelectric effect 30–31, 33
computed radiography (CR) 34, 34–37, 41
  Appendix notes 279
  quality assurance 55–58

cone beam artefact 108
contrast (agent)
  in digital subtraction angiography (DSA) 72, 73
  in MR imaging 188, 190–191
  in ultrasound 121, 212
contrast-enhanced ultrasound (CEUS) 212
contrast (image quality) 43, 50–51
  image contrast 44–45, 51, 101, 246–247
  subject contrast 43–44, 50–51, 101, 246
controlled areas (designated under IRR17) 268
cooling chart, anode 20
count density 246
CT (computerised tomography) imaging 77–111
  Appendix notes 283–284
  artefacts 103–109
  axial scanning 85
  dose 110–111, 275–276
  dual-energy CT (DECT) 93–96
  electron beam scanner 83
  equipment 79–84, 87–88
  hybrid SPECT/CT 236
  image processing 90–92
  image quality 97–102
  multislice scanning 86–88, 108
  pitch 86, 88
  rotate-fixed scanner 83
  rotate-rotate scanner 82
  spiral/helical scanning 85, 107
  translate-rotate scanner 81–82
CTDI (CT dose index) 110–111, 275–276
CT number (CT number (Hounsfield Units)) 45, 90–92
cupping artefact 104
cyclotron production of radioisotopes 215

D

damping 123
DAP (dose area product) 293. See also diagnostic reference levels (DRLs)
DECT (dual-energy CT) imaging 93–96
dental radiology 18
depth of view, in ultrasound imaging 124
detective quantum efficiency (DQE) 37, 52, 279
detector array, in CT imaging 80–81, 87–88, 98
detector dose indicator (DDI) 55–56
detector, in gamma camera 226–227
deterministic vs stochastic effects of radiation 261–262
diagnostic reference levels (DRLs) 264–265
diffusion coefficient 177
  apparent diffusion coefficient (ADC) 178

diffusion tensor imaging, in MR imaging 179
diffusion weighted imaging, in MR imaging
    177–181
digital enhancement of x-ray images 37
digital image processing and enhancement.
        See image processing and enhancement
digital radiography (DR) 34, 37–40, 41–42
    Appendix notes 279
    quality assurance 55–58
digital subtraction angiography (DSA) 72
display. See image display
distortion artefacts
    in MR imaging 196–198
    in x-ray imaging 50
Doppler angle 133
Doppler, in ultrasound 119, 130
    artefacts 132–133
    colour Doppler 131, 132
    continuous wave doppler 130
    power Doppler 131
    pulsed wave Doppler 130–132
    spectral Doppler 131–132
dose area product (DAP) 293. See also diagnostic
        reference levels (DRLs)
dose, radiation
    and x-ray beam properties 275
    Appendix notes 292
    diagnostic reference levels (DRLs) 264–265
    entrance skin/surface dose (ESD) 72
    equivalent dose. See equivalent dose
    and filter use 275
    in fluoroscopy 68, 72–73, 275
    in CT 110–111, 275–276
    in nuclear medicine 276
    legislation. See Ionising Radiation Regulations
        2017 (IRR17)
    limits per calendar year 267
    in mammography 62
    measurement 260–261
    and noise 48
    overexposure 268
    and patient properties 275, 276
    and rectification 22
    to staff 73. See also radiation protection
    vs contrast 60
dose, x-ray
    effective dose (E). See effective dose (E)
dosimetry badges 273–274
DQE (detective quantum efficiency) 37, 52, 279
dual-energy CT imaging 93–96
dynamic range, of detectors 36, 41, 80

echo-planar imaging (EPI) 177–178, 200
echo train length (ETL), in MR imaging 171–172,
    172
edge ringing artefact, in MR imaging 200
edge unsharpness 49–50
effective dose (E) 111, 260–261. See also dose,
        radiation
    Appendix notes 296–297
    average, from background radiation 259
    limits 267
effective focal spot 18, 19, 20. See also focusing,
        x-ray
elastic scatter (Rayleigh scattering) 30
electromagnetic (EM) radiation 6–9
    as particles 6–7. See also photons
    as waves 6, 278
electromagnetic spectrum 8
electron capture 13, 14
electronic dosimeters 274–276
electron optics, in image intensifier system 68
electrons 3, 3–4. See also beta particles
    auger electrons 11
    bound and free electrons 4
    shells 3–4
electrostatic force, in nucleus 4–5
endocrine imaging 220
energy fluence 7
energy fluence rate 7
energy resolution, in nuclear medicine 255
enhancement. See image processing and en-
        hancement
entrance skin dose (entrance surface dose)
        (ESD) 72
Environmental Permitting Regulations 2016 (EPR
        16) 269
equivalent dose 260. See also dose, radiation
    limits 267
ESD (entrance skin/surface dose) 72
exposure index (EI) (speed) 36, 52
exposure time, x-ray 19, 20, 22

fat saturation artefact 198–199
fat/water cancellation artefact 198
fibre tracking map 179
field of view (FOV), in MR imaging 193
filament 17, 18. See also thermionic emission
    filament current 22
fill factor, in DR 38

film badges 273
filters, in MR imaging 166–167
filtration, in nuclear medicine 234, 239, 250
filtration, in x-ray imaging 17, 20
  and x-ray spectrum 25
  "bow-tie" filter 79, 104
  in CT imaging 79, 104, 105
  in mammography 60–61
  and patient dose 275
FLAIR (FLuid Attenuated Inversion Recovery)
    sequence 175, 176
flat panel detector 71–72
flow void artefact 186, 188
fluence, energy 7
fluence, photon 7, 100
fluorescence 213
fluorescence, x-ray 34–35
fluorography 65, 71
fluoroscopy 19
  accelerating potential 21
  Appendix notes 280
  definitions 65
  dose 68, 72–73, 275
  equipment configuration 66
  image display 69–70
  image intensifier (and system). See image inten-
    sifier (II)
  magnification 68
  minimising staff dose 271
focal spot 18, 48, 50, 61
  in CT imaging 98
  quality assurance 55
  size 19, 20, 48, 52, 55, 61, 64, 98
focal track 18
focus-detector distance (FDD)
  in mammography 59
focusing, ultrasound 125
focusing, x-ray
  focal spot 18, 19, 20
  focusing cup 17, 18
Fourier Transformation (FT) 161, 248
fractional anisotropy (FA) map 179
frequency encoding, in MR imaging 160–161

G

gain calibration 39
gallbladder imaging 232
gamma camera 225–231
  collimator 225–226, 232–233, 237
  detector 226–227
  image display 229, 234
  image formation 227–229, 232–234

image processing 234–235, 239
  malfunction 252
  planar imaging 232–235
  quality assurance 254–255
  spatial resolution 249
  SPECT imaging 236–239, 252–253, 255
gamma particles 11
  decay model 13
gantry, in CT imaging 81, 85
gastrointestinal (GI) imaging 221, 232
geometric unsharpness 48–49, 52
ghost images 37
Gibbs artefact, in MR imaging 200
glass envelope, in x-ray tube 17, 20
gradient coils, in MR imaging 140
gradient (recalled) echo (GRE) sequence, in MR
    imaging 173–174, 187
grey-scale modification
  in digital radiography 40
  in fluoroscopy 71
grids
  anti-scatter grids 44, 59, 61
  and fluoroscopy 275
  grid cut-off 50
  and mammography 59, 61
  and Moiré patterns 37
  and patient dose 275

H

half-life, of radiopharmaceuticals 215, 216, 219,
    220, 221, 289
half value layer (HVL) 31
harmonics, in ultrasound imaging 128
head scan (CT) 103
heating, anode 19, 20
heel effect, anode 20, 59
helical artefacts, in CT imaging 107
hepatic imaging 95
"herringbone" artefact, in MR imaging 199
Hounsfield Units 45, 90–92
HVL (half value layer) 31
hydrogen nuclei, as magnets 141

I

ICNIRP 202, 203, 204
image density in x-ray imaging 37
image display
  gamma camera display 229, 234
  monitors and hardcopy 40
  windowing 45, 60, 229, 234
image intensifier (II) 65–69

brightness gain 65–66
and noise 48
image processing and enhancement
in digital radiography (DR) 40
in CT imaging 90–92
in fluoroscopy 71
in nuclear medicine 234–235, 239, 244
image quality. See also artefacts in MR imaging;
artefacts in nuclear medicine; artefacts
in ultrasound imaging; artefacts in x-ray
imaging
Appendix notes 280–281, 291
in computed radiography (CR) 36–37, 56–58
contrast. See contrast (image quality)
CT imaging 97–102
in direct radiography (DR) 39–40, 56–58
fluoroscopy 70–71
gamma camera 228, 229
magnification 49–50, 50
noise. See noise (signal)
nuclear medicine 228, 229, 246–251
quality assurance testing 56–58
resolution. See spatial resolution
screen-film radiography (SCR)
screen-film 36
unsharpness 48–49
image receptor unsharpness 52
incomplete projection, in CT imaging 105, 107
infants, MR imaging 203
infection/inflammation imaging 220
inherent scatter. See Compton effect (Compton
scatter)
Institute of Physics and Engineering in Medicine
(IPEM) report 91 53
intensity. See also attenuation; contrast (image
quality); spatial resolution;
energy fluence rate 7
intensity
of sound wave 116
inverse square law 8
of sound wave 123
photon energy 6
internal conversion 11
International Commission on Non-Ionizing Radiation Protection (ICNIRP) 202, 203, 204
International Electrotechnical Commission (IEC)
202
inverse square law 7, 7–8
inversion recovery sequence, in MR imaging
175–176
iodine
k-edge and tissue contrast 30
ionisation chamber detector, in CT imaging

80–81
ionising radiation. See also radiation protection
dose. See dose, radiation
effects 261–263
types and sources 259
Ionising Radiation (Medical Exposure) Regulations
2017 (IR(ME))R 2017) 264–265, 268, 269
Ionising Radiation Regulations 2017 (IRR17) 254,
266–268
isomeric transition 13, 14
isomers 10
isotones 10
isotopes 10
iterative reconstruction, in CT imaging 92

K

k-edge and l-edge (photoelectric effect) 29–30,
60, 93
kinetic energy, of electrons 4
K-Space, in MR imaging 166–167

L

LAC (linear attenuation coefficient). See linear
attenuation coefficient (LAC)
Larmor frequency 141–142, 144, 157, 182
latitude. See dynamic range, of detectors
linear attenuation coefficient (LAC) 31, 44, 90–92
photoelectric linear attenuation coefficient 29
linear energy transfer (LET) 260
luminescence. See bioluminescence; thermoluminescent detectors (TLDs); x-ray luminescence (fluorescence and phosphorescence)
lung imaging 220, 232

M

MAC (mass attenuation coefficient) 31–32
magnetic saturation, in MR angiography 185
magnetism, types of 190
magnification 49–50, 50
mammography 21, 59–64
Appendix notes 279
tomosynthesis 62–63
mask algorithm, in spatial feature enhancement
40
mask images
and digital subtraction angiography (DSA) 72
and gain calibration 39–40
mass attenuation coefficient (MAC) 31–32

mass number 3
matrix
  in MR imaging 192–193
  in SPECT imaging 237
mechanical coefficient (Q-value) 124–123
mechanical index (MI) 121
Medicines and Healthcare Products Regulatory
      Agency (MHRA) 202, 204
metabolites, and MR spectroscopy (MRS)
      182–183
metallic artefacts 106, 180
metal related hazards, in MR imaging 205
MHRA 202, 204
microwave heating, in MR imaging 203–204
mirror/reflection artefact, in ultrasound imaging
      135
misregistration 72
M-mode (ultrasound) 119
mobile radiography 19
modulation transfer function (MTF) 37, 46
Moiré patterns 37
molecular imaging
  Appendix notes 289–291
  contrast-enhanced ultrasound (CEUS) 212
  introduction and definitions 211
  MR spectroscopy. See MR spectroscopy (MRS)
  non-nuclear molecular imaging. See con-
     trast-enhanced ultrasound (CEUS); optical
     imaging (bioluminescence and fluores-
     cence)
  nuclear medicine (NM). See nuclear medicine
     (NM)
  optical imaging (bioluminescence and fluores-
     cence) 212–213
movement unsharpness/motion artefacts 49,
      106, 196, 247, 249
  flow void artefact 186, 188
MR angiography 185–189
  Appendix notes 287
  flow effects 185–187
  techniques 187–189
MR (magnetic resonance) imaging
  angiography. See MR angiography
  Appendix notes 286–288, 295
  artefacts 161–162, 179–180, 186, 188, 196–201
  contraindications 205–206
  contrast agents 188, 190–191
  diffusion tensor imaging 179
  diffusion weighted imaging 177–181
  echo-planar imaging (EPI) 177–178, 200
  emergencies 206
  fast advanced spin echo (HASTE) sequence
     172, 201

filters 166–167
frequency encoding 160–163, 168
gradient (recalled) echo (GRE) sequence
     173–174, 187
image quality 192–195
inversion recovery sequence 175–176
K-Space 166–167
MR machine 139–140
MR physics (introduction) 141–143
multi echo sequence 171
multi slice sequence 170–171
phase encoding 164–165, 168, 169
proton density (PD) imaging 153–154, 154
relaxation. See relaxation, in MR imaging
safety issues 202–207
slice selection 157–159, 168, 193–194
spatial encoding (introduction) 155–156
spectroscopy. See MR spectroscopy (MRS)
spin echo sequence 148–150, 168–172, 177–178
T1 and T2 signal 144–147
T1-weighted imaging 151–152, 154
T2-weighted imaging 152–153, 154
turbo spin echo (TSE) sequence 171–172
MR spectroscopy (MRS) 182–184
  Appendix notes 286–287
MTF (modulation transfer function) 37, 46
multi echo sequence, in MR imaging 171
multi slice sequence, in MR imaging 170–171
multi-voxel chemical shift imaging (CSI) 183

N

neutrinos 12
neutrons 3, 4–5, 13
noise (acoustic), in MR imaging 205
noise (signal) 47–48, 51
  in CT imaging 100–101
  measurement 100
  in MR imaging 194
  in nuclear medicine 247, 249–250
  signal-to-noise ratio (SNR) 194, 233
nuclear bombardment production of radioiso-
     topes 215
nuclear medicine
  PET imaging. See PET imaging (positron emis-
     sion tomography)
nuclear medicine (NM)
  and breast feeding 263, 272
  Appendix notes 289–291, 295
  artefacts 238, 239, 252–253
  dose 276
  gamma camera. See gamma camera
  image processing 234–235, 239, 244

image quality 228, 229, 246–251
planar imaging 232–235
quality assurance 254–255
radioisotope production 215–218
radiopharmaceuticals 219–224, 241, 252, 289
regulations 269
SPECT imaging 236–239, 252–253, 255
nuclear reactor production of radioisotopes
        215–216
nucleons. See neutrons; protons
nucleus 3
nuclear stability 4–5, 10–11
nuclides 10, 11
Nyquist frequency/limit 47, 132, 161

oncological imaging
CT imaging 95
nuclear medicine (NM) 220
ophthalmology 119, 121
optical density. See contrast (image quality)
optical imaging (bioluminescence and fluores-
        cence) 212–213
overexposure, reporting 268

pair production 70
partial volume artefact 104
patient dosimetry 275–276. See also dose, radia-
        tion; radiation protection
penumbra 48, 50. See also unsharpness
perfused blood volume imaging 95
PET imaging (positron emission tomography)
        240–245
Appendix notes 291
image quality 249–250
phantom
CT imaging 100, 108, 110
nuclear medicine 254, 254–255
x-ray imaging 55
phased array, in MR imaging 140
phase encoding, in MR imaging 164–165, 168,
        169
phosphorescence, x-ray 34–35
photocathode 67, 227
photoconductor, in digital radiography (DR) 39
photoelectric effect 28–30, 93
vs Compton effect 30–31, 33
photoelectric linear attenuation coefficient (LAC).
        See also linear attenuation coefficient (LAC)

photomultiplier tubes (PMT), in gamma camera
        227
photon fluence 7, 100
photons 6–8
photon starvation, in CT imaging 105–106
piezoelectric effect 123–124
piezoelectric material 120, 123
pitch, in CT imaging 86, 88
pixel-calibration 40
pixels 36, 90, 91, 192, 233
pixel size 99, 100, 249
planar imaging, in nuclear medicine 232–235
positron-electron annihilation 240–241
positron emission (beta plus decay) 12, 240
positron emission tomography (PET). See PET
        imaging (positron emission tomography)
positron range 250
precession, in MR imaging 141–142, 143, 144
pregnancy
and MR imaging 203, 206
radiation-related risks 262–263
staff, and radiation protection 272
and ultrasound imaging 121, 130
primary and secondary radiation (and radiation
        protection) 270–271
principal diffusion direction map 179
proton density (PD) imaging, in MR imaging
        153–154, 154
protons 3, 10
Pulsatility Index (PI) 132
pulse repetition frequency (PRF), in ultrasound
        imaging 124, 128–127

quality assurance (QA)
Appendix notes 281–282
nuclear medicine 254–255
x-ray imaging 53–58
quality, image. See image quality
quantum mottle 247
Q-value (mechanical coefficient) 124–123

radiation, ionising. See ionising radiation
radiation protection. See also dose, radiation; ion-
        ising radiation
Appendix notes 292–295
dosimetry badges 273–274
legislation 264–269
minimising staff dose 73, 271–272
roles and responsibilities 265, 266

sources of radiation 270–271
radiation risk assessment 266
radioactive decay 10–14
   decay models 11, 12–13
   types of radiation 11–12
radioisotope production
   cyclotron (nuclear bombardment) 215
   nuclear reactor 215–216
   radionuclide generator 216–217
radionuclides 10, 13
radiopharmaceuticals 219–224, 241, 252, 289
radiotherapy 18
Rayleigh scattering 30
read-out gradient, in MR imaging 160–161
rectification 21–22, 26
reflection, of sound waves 117
refraction, of sound waves 117
region of interest (ROI) analysis, in nuclear medi-
      cine 234
regulatory bodies 202, 203
relaxation, in MR imaging 143
   Spin-Lattice/Longitudinal Relaxation (T1 Recov-
      ery) 143, 145, 147
   Spin-Spin Relaxation (T2 Decay) 143, 146–147,
      147
renal imaging
   CT imaging 95
   nuclear medicine 220, 232
Resistive Index (RI) 131–132
resolution. See spatial resolution
resonance
   in MR imaging 142
   in ultrasound imaging 123
resonant antenna effect, in MR imaging 205
reverberation artefact, in ultrasound imaging
      134–135
RF artefacts, in MR imaging 199
RF fields in MR imaging, safety issues 203–204
RF (radiofrequency) coils, in MR imaging 140,
      199
ring artefact, in CT imaging 107
ring down artefact, in ultrasound imaging 135
rotating anode 19

S

sampling pitch/frequency
   in digital detectors 47
   in MR imaging 161
   in ultrasound imaging 132
scatter
   anti-scatter grids 44, 59, 61
   coincidence, in PET imaging 243

Compton scatter. See Compton effect (Compton
      scatter)
   and contrast 44
   elastic scatter (Rayleigh scattering) 30
   rejection, in gamma camera 228
   sound waves 118
scintillation crystals (detectors)
   in digital radiography (DR) 38
   in gamma camera 226, 228
   in PET imaging 241
screen-film radiography (SFR) 34, 36
secondary radiation (and radiation protection)
      270–271
Segré chart for nuclear stability 5, 10
sensitivity number (SI) 36
shielding (radiation protection) 271–272
shim coils, in MR imaging 139
signal-to-noise ratio (SNR) 194, 233. See
      also noise (signal)
single photon emission computed tomography
      (SPECT) 236–239, 252–253, 255
single voxel spectroscopy (SVS) 183
slice selection, in MR imaging 157–159, 168,
      193–194
SNR (signal-to-noise ratio) 194, 233. See
      also noise (signal)
solid state detector (SSD), in CT imaging 80
sonogram 131
sound waves. See also ultrasound imaging
   attenuation 116–118
   characteristics 115–116
   interaction with tissue 116–118
   vs electromagnetic radiation 115
spatial filtering, in fluoroscopy 71
spatial resolution 51
   Appendix notes 296
   in computed radiography (CR) 36–37
   in CT imaging 97–100
   and digital detector properties 46–47, 48, 52
   factors affecting 46
   in fluoroscopy 71
   in mammography 61
   measurement 45
   in MR imaging 192–194
   in nuclear medicine 233, 248–249, 250, 254
   in ultrasound 127
specific absorption ratio (SAR) 203–204
SPECT imaging (single photon emission comput-
      ed tomography) 236–239, 252–253, 255
spectral broadening, in ultrasound imaging 132
spectroscopy, MR. See MR spectroscopy (MRS)
speed (exposure index) 36, 52
spin echo sequence, in MR imaging 148–150,

168–172, 177–178
star artefact 239
stationary anode 18
steady state free precession (SSFP) imaging 201
STIR (Short Tau Inversion Recovery) sequence
 175
stochastic vs deterministic effects of radiation
 261–262
streak artefact
 and incomplete projection 105, 107
 and photon starvation 105–106
strong nuclear force 4–5
subject contrast 43–44, 50–51, 101, 246
supervised area (designated under IRR17) 268

T

T1 and T2, in MR imaging 144–147, 151–152,
 152–153, 154
T2 dark-through artefact 179
T2 shine-through artefact 179
target (in x-ray tube) 17, 18. See also anode
 atomic number, and x-ray spectrum 26
 in mammography 60–61
 target angle 19, 20
temporal filtering, in fluoroscopy 71
temporal resolution, in ultrasound imaging
 127–128
testing equipment. See quality assurance (QA)
TFT (thin-film transistor) array, in digital radiography (DR) 38
thermal index (TI) 120–121
thermionic emission 17, 18, 21–22. See also cathode; filament; x-ray production
thermoluminescent detectors (TLDs) 273–274
time activity curves, in nuclear medicine 235
time to echo (TE), in MR imaging 149, 152–153,
 171
 effective time to echo (Teff) 172
time to repetition (TR), in MR imaging 150, 151,
 152, 170, 187
tissue weighting factor 261
tomography. See CT (computerised tomography)
 imaging; PET imaging (positron emission
 tomography); SPECT imaging (single photon emission computed tomography)
tomosynthesis 62–63
transaxial resolution, in CT imaging 97–99
transverse magnetisation, in MR imaging 142–
 143, 143
tube current 22
 modulation 106
 and x-ray spectrum 25

tube potential, and x-ray spectrum 25
tube rating 19
turbo spin echo (TSE) sequence, in MR imaging
 171–172
TV camera tube, in fluoroscopy 69

U

ultrasound imaging 113–135
 Appendix notes 285
 artefacts 128, 132–133, 134–135
 beam focus 125
 B-Mode transducer 119–120
 compound imaging 129
 contrast-enhanced ultrasound (CEUS) 212
 depth of view 124
 Doppler. See Doppler, in ultrasound
 harmonics 128
 modes 119, 123
 piezoelectric effect 123–124
 in pregnancy 121, 130
 pulse duration 123
 pulse repetition frequency (PRF) 124, 128–127
 safety issues 120–121, 128
 spatial resolution 127
 temporal resolution 127–128
 transducer array 124–125
 ultrasound frequency 115
unsharpness 48–49

V

vascular imaging 95, 128, 131–132, 133, 232. See
 also MR angiography
vignetting 72
virtual non-calcium imaging 95
virtual unenhanced imaging 95
voxels, in MRS 183–184

W

wall filters, in ultrasound imaging 133
windowing 45, 60, 229, 234
window, in x-ray tube 17, 20, 67, 69

X

x-ray attenuation 27
 and beam quality 32, 93
 Compton effect. See Compton effect (Compton
 scatter)
 elastic scatter (Rayleigh scattering) 30
 factors affecting 30–31
 and image contrast 43–44

linear attenuation coefficient. *See* linear attenuation coefficient (LAC)
    measurement 31–32
    and noise 48
    photoelectric effect. *See* photoelectric effect
x-ray beam angle 50
x-ray beam heterogeneity 32
x-ray beam width, and attenuation 32
x-ray equipment 17, 18–21
    automatic exposure control (AEC). *See* automatic exposure control (AEC) (in fluorography and radiography)
    computed radiography (CT) 34–35
    digital radiography (DR) 38–39
    image intensifier. *See* image intensifier (II)
    mammography 59–61, 62
    other components 20–21
    testing 53–58
x-ray imaging
    Appendix notes 279–282
    computed radiography (CR). *See* computed radiography (CR)
    digital radiography (DR). *See* digital radiography (DR)
    fluoroscopy. *See* fluoroscopy
    screen-film radiography (SFR) 34, 36
x-ray luminescence (fluorescence and phosphorescence) 34–35
x-ray production 17–26
x-ray spectrum 24, 24–26
x-ray tube. *See also* x-ray production
    anode. *See* anode
    cathode. *See* cathode
    image intensifier system 67–69
    tube current. *See* tube current
    tube current, and x-ray spectrum 25
    tube potential, and x-ray spectrum 25
    tube rating 19

Z

Z-sensitivity, in CT scanning 99–100
Z value, in gamma camera 227–228

We welcome your feedback so please feel free to contact us via the website www.radiologycafe.com, or alternatively you can follow us on social media.

Twitter   : **@radiologycafe**
Facebook : **facebook.com/radiologycafe**
Linkedin   : **linkedin.com/company/radiology-cafe**
Instagram : **@radiology.cafe**

We hope you found these revision notes useful!

Dr Sarah Abdulla
Dr Christopher Clarke

Lightning Source UK Ltd.
Milton Keynes UK
UKHW050454230922
409307UK00002B/115

* 9 7 8 1 9 9 9 9 8 8 5 2 4 *